INTERDISCIPLINARITY AND WELLBEING

In this book, the authors provide a much-needed general theory of interdisciplinarity and relate it to health/wellbeing research and professional practice. In so doing they make it possible for practitioners of the different disciplines to communicate without contradiction or compromise, resolving the tensions that beset much interdisciplinary work.

Such a general theory is only possible if we assume that there is more to being (ontology) than empirical being (what we can measure directly). Therefore, the unique approach to interdisciplinarity applied in this book starts from ontology, namely that there is a multimechanismicity (a multiplicity of mechanisms) in open systems, and then moves to epistemology. By contrast, the mainstream approach, which fails to acknowledge ontology, is "unserious" and tends to result in a methodological hierarchy, unconducive of interdisciplinarity, in which empiricist science is overtly or tacitly assumed to be the superior version of science.

This book is primarily aimed at those people interested in improving health and wellbeing – such as researchers, policy-makers, educators, and general practitioners. However, it will also be useful to academics engaged in the broader academic debate on interdisciplinary metatheory.

Roy Bhaskar was the originator of the philosophy of critical realism and the author of many acclaimed and influential works including *A Realist Theory of Science* (1975); *The Possibility of Naturalism* (1979); *Scientific Realism and Human Emancipation* (1986); *Reclaiming Reality* (1989); *Philosophy and the Idea of Freedom* (1991); *Dialectic: The Pulse of Freedom* (1993); *Reflections on Meta-Reality* (2002); and *From Science to Emancipation* (2011).

Berth Danermark is Professor Emeritus of Sociology at the School of Health Sciences, Örebro University, Sweden. He is also the Director of Doctoral Studies (and founder member) of the Swedish Institute of Disability Research.

Leigh Price is Senior Research Associate at the Environmental Learning and Research Centre, Rhodes University, South Africa, and Editor of the *Journal of Critical Realism*.

ROUTLEDGE STUDIES IN CRITICAL REALISM

Some other books in the series:

Maurice Mandelbaum and American Critical Realism
Edited by Ian Verstegen

Contributions to Social Ontology
Edited by Clive Lawson, John Spiro Latsis, and Nuno Miguel Ornelin Martins

Critical Realism, Post-positivism and the Possibility of Knowledge
By Ruth Groff

Emergentist Marxism
Dialectical Philosophy and Social Theory
By Sean Creaven

Engendering the State
The International Diffusion of Women's Human Rights
By Lynn Savery

Explaining Global Poverty
A Critical Realist Approach
By Branwen Gruffydd Jones

Ontology of Sex
By Carrie Hull

Revitalizing Causality
Realism about Causality in Philosophy and Social Science
Edited by Ruth Groff

Interdisciplinarity and Wellbeing
A Critical Realist General Theory of Interdisciplinarity
By Roy Bhaskar, Berth Danermark, and Leigh Price

INTERDISCIPLINARITY AND WELLBEING

A Critical Realist General Theory of Interdisciplinarity

Roy Bhaskar, Berth Danermark, and Leigh Price

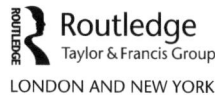

LONDON AND NEW YORK

First published 2018
by Routledge
2 Park Square, Milton Park, Abingdon, Oxon OX14 4RN

and by Routledge
711 Third Avenue, New York, NY 10017

Routledge is an imprint of the Taylor & Francis Group, an informa business

© 2018 Roy Bhaskar, Berth Danermark, and Leigh Price

The right of Roy Bhaskar, Berth Danermark, and Leigh Price to be identified as authors of this work has been asserted by them in accordance with sections 77 and 78 of the Copyright, Designs and Patents Act 1988.

All rights reserved. No part of this book may be reprinted or reproduced or utilized in any form or by any electronic, mechanical, or other means, now known or hereafter invented, including photocopying and recording, or in any information storage or retrieval system, without permission in writing from the publishers.

Trademark notice: Product or corporate names may be trademarks or registered trademarks, and are used only for identification and explanation without intent to infringe.

British Library Cataloguing in Publication Data
A catalogue record for this book is available from the British Library

Library of Congress Cataloging in Publication Data
A catalog record for this book has been requested

ISBN: 978-0-415-40371-9 (hbk)
ISBN: 978-0-415-49666-7 (pbk)
ISBN: 978-1-315-17729-8 (ebk)

Typeset in Bembo
by Taylor & Francis Books

CONTENTS

List of illustrations	*vii*
Foreword	*viii*
Acknowledgements	*x*
List of acronyms	*xi*
1 Introduction	1

PART I
Antinomies of mainstream interdisciplinarity · 7

2 Overview of the contemporary literature	9
3 Contemporary ways to justify interdisciplinarity	15

PART II
A critical realist general theory of interdisciplinarity · 21

4 Core concepts of critical realism	23
5 Critical realism and social science	32
6 The ontological case for interdisciplinarity	44
7 The seven steps to deeper understanding of ontology	54
8 Critical realism and the alternative metatheories/methodologies	74

PART III
Applied interdisciplinary research — 83

9 Biophysical interventions are not enough: the hidden (holistic) healing ensemble — 85

10 The seven enigmas of healing — 89

11 The biopsychosocial approach, with special reference to the International Classification of Functioning, Disability and Health — 113

12 The practical organization of interdisciplinary co-operation — 123

13 Understanding methodological imperialism — 131

14 Interdisciplinarity in action: explaining the epidemiology of HIV — 137

15 Concluding considerations — 148

References — *157*
Index — *168*

ILLUSTRATIONS

Figures

5.1	Social life and wellbeing in the context of four-planar social being	35
10.1	Transformist politics	110
11.1	The biopsychosocial framework of the ICF	116
11.2	The phases in the development of the ICF core sets	120
12.1	Phases in the achievement of interdisciplinarity	124
14.1	Findings from literature review theorizing the HIV situation in southern Africa	138

Tables

2.1	Dimensions, problems, and conditions related to interdisciplinarity	14
6.1	Examples of critical realist interpretations of laminated systems	49
10.1	An interdisciplinary explanation for the causal mechanisms of diabetes	98
10.2	Examples of mechanisms relevant to anorexia at different levels of reality	109
12.1	Recommendations from the literature for successful interdisciplinarity	129

FOREWORD

Ten years ago, when Roy Bhaskar was a guest professor at the Swedish Institute of Disability Research at Örebro University, we collaborated on a paper (Bhaskar and Danermark, 2006) that looked at interdisciplinary research from a critical realist perspective. After writing this paper, Roy Bhaskar became increasingly aware of the significant contribution that applied critical realism could make to interdisciplinary research, and consequently the idea for this book was born. Some years later, in 2012, we invited Leigh Price to join us. At the time, she was working with Roy Bhaskar as a Visiting Research Associate at the Institute of Education, University College London, and she had written several papers that demonstrated the value of using critical realism to guide interdisciplinarity.

Sadly, Roy Bhaskar passed away before this book was finished. However, his contributions to the introduction and conclusion were by this time written; and we had from the start planned to base the section outlining critical realism on lectures that he had presented while delivering a course in critical realism at The University College of Oslo, Norway. Leigh Price, in consultation with Berth Danermark, converted these lectures to chapters, attempting to remain as faithful to Roy's original meaning as possible. However, considerable changes had to be made to the text to achieve an accessible style. Readers should also note that the introduction refers to certain phrases such as "polymorphous presence" which would usually be mentioned again, elsewhere in the text, but in this case Roy passed away before the rest of the book was written. Although this book is in many ways an exemplar of collaboration, making it at times difficult to distinguish between particular contributions, special mention should be given to Chapters 9 and 10, where Berth and Leigh develop Roy's concepts of the *hidden (holistic) holistic ensemble* and the *seven enigmas of healing*. Berth was lead author in Chapters 2, 11, 12, and 13; and Leigh was lead author in Chapters 3 and 14. Roy read and commented on early versions, or at least the outlines, of these chapters. If we leave aside questions of interpretation, Chapters 4 to 8 are mainly the work of Roy, as conveyed in his Oslo lectures, with exceptions being his collaboration with Berth on interdisciplinarity (indicated in the text) and the addition of several illustrative examples by Leigh. All three authors made contributions to the introduction. The conclusion was written by Berth and Leigh, although echoes of Roy's voice come through strongly. The outline of critical realism that we provide in this book is designed to support our main objective, which is to explain how to carry out interdisciplinary work. Therefore, if readers want to understand critical realism more deeply, or if they have questions about how Roy came to certain understandings, we encourage them to refer to his earlier works, such as *A Realist Theory of Science* (2008a/1975), *The Possibility of Naturalism* (2014/1979), *Scientific Realism and Human Emancipation* (2009/1986), *Dialectic: The Pulse of Freedom* (2008b/1993), and *The Philosophy of MetaReality: Creativity, Love and Freedom* (2012/2002).

Berth Danermark and Leigh Price
January 2017

ACKNOWLEDGEMENTS

We would like to thank our various institutions for their loyalty over the years: namely, the Institute of Education, University College London; the Swedish Institute of Disability Research at Örebro University; and the Environmental Learning Research Centre, Rhodes University, South Africa. Leigh Price would like to thank the Sandisa Mbewu Fund for financing her post-doctoral fellowship at Rhodes University, and Heila Lotz Sisitka for her invaluable practical and intellectual support. She would also like to thank Jane Gair for her unfaltering encouragement. We are grateful to Cheryl Frank, who carefully transcribed Roy's lectures. She regrettably passed away in 2010, but we sincerely thank her posthumously. We feel confident that if Roy were still with us, he would thank Rebecca Long and Hilary Wainwright. We would also like to thank Rae and Jan Vermeulen for their helpful comments on certain of the chapters.

ACRONYMS

ADHD	Attention Deficit Hyperactivity Disorder
AIDS	Acquired Immune Deficiency Syndrome
BMJ	*British Medical Journal*
CA(I)MO	Context, Agent, social Intervention, Mechanism, Outcome
DEA	Diagnosis, Explanation, Action
DREI(C)	Description, Retroduction, Elimination, Identification, and Correction
DSM	Diagnostic and Statistical Manual of Mental Disorders
EMR	Electromagnetic Radiation
EURAB	European Union Research Advisory Board
HIV	Human Immunodeficiency Virus
ICF	International Classification of Functioning, Disability and Health
MELD	first Moment, second Edge, third Level, fourth Dimension
NAS	National Academy of Sciences
PHL	Person with Hearing Loss
QOF	Quality and Outcomes Framework
RCT	Randomized Controlled Trial
RRREI(C)	Resolution, Redescription, Retroduction, Elimination, Identification, Correction
RRRIREI(C)	Resolution, Redescription, Retroduction, Inference to best explanation, Retroduction, Elimination, Identification of antecedents, Correction
TINA	There Is No Alternative
TMSA	Transformational Model of Social Activity
TTTTTT	Transformed, Transformative, Trustworthy, Totalizing, Transformist, Transitional
UNAIDS	Joint United Nations Programme on HIV/AIDS
WHO	World Health Organisation

1
INTRODUCTION

Many of the major players in health and wellbeing research have made multi- and interdisciplinary research a priority. These include: the World Health Organization (1986), as stated in *The Ottawa Charter*; and the European Commission (2014), as stated in *Horizon 2020*, a framework for health research and technology. In the fields of health and wellbeing, this acknowledged need for interdisciplinarity is often framed as a call for interventions guided by the biopsychosocial model, originally developed by George Engel in 1977. However, as we explain in the section on the antinomies of contemporary interdisciplinarity, despite the extravagant lip service paid to interdisciplinarity, there is little sophisticated analysis in the literature that explains its philosophical necessity. Neither can it be said that interdisciplinarity has, to date, been an unqualified success. In this book, we aim to repair these shortcomings by addressing two overriding questions:

1. Why is interdisciplinarity necessary?
2. How is it possible in practice?

To answer these questions, we approach interdisciplinarity from the perspective of ontology, using a critical realist epistemology. For example, we suggest how sophisticated research procedures can be designed to enable scientists to integrate the knowledge gained from various individual disciplines. This metatheoretical approach avoids unilinear reductionism, additive atomism, and naïve eclecticism alike. We also discuss the practical issues involved in achieving interdisciplinarity, such as how to encourage co-operation among researchers. We answer the question asked by some – whether there should be disciplines at all – with a resounding "yes". This is because the complexity required by interdisciplinarity is best achieved by an efficient division of labour, enabled by well-defined disciplines with clearly differentiated tasks. However, the existence of well-defined disciplines does not prevent the transdisciplinary processes that eventually transcend the disciplines and result in interdisciplinarity.

The essence of our argument is that the need for interdisciplinarity is an unavoidable consequence of the open-systemic character within which practically all events occur. Critical realists, the present authors included, have begun to theorize the concepts essential for the understanding of interdisciplinary work in this open system context, such as stratification and emergence, absence and contradiction, internal relationality and holistic causality (see e.g. Bhaskar and Danermark, 2006; Høyer and Naess, 2008; Bhaskar et al., 2010; Holland, 2014; Price 2014a). However, there is, to date, no major treatment within the critical realist genre exploring the rationale or implications of the necessity for interdisciplinary work.

Finkenthal (2001) posed the question: "What makes interdisciplinarity possible and/or desirable?" This question can be addressed from at least three perspectives. The first, and probably the most common, is from a practical perspective, for instance, how to educate students in interdisciplinary research and how to nurture interdisciplinary milieus. The second perspective is epistemological and focuses on the conditions, possibilities, nature, and limits of knowledge production that stems from interdisciplinarity, for instance this perspective considers the challenges faced by researchers when they attempt to integrate elements in the interdisciplinary process. A third perspective is to bring ontological questions – that is, questions about reality – to the fore. From this perspective, the question posed by Finkenthal can be sharpened and becomes, "What must the nature of reality be like for interdisciplinarity to be possible, and necessary, and such a strikingly pervasive (and talked about) feature of our experience?"

Therefore, in this book, our argument for interdisciplinarity starts from ontology, namely, multimechanismicity (a multiplicity of mechanisms) in open systems; and moves to epistemology, namely multidisciplinarity, interdisciplinarity, intradisciplinarity, crossdisciplinarity, and transdisciplinarity. We assume the presence of a *necessary laminated system*, which is a stratified totality, constituted by emergent levels. Any explanation will need reference to each level, hence the need for antireductionism and interdisciplinarity alike. The necessary laminated system involves an internal relation between the levels or elements of a system, constituting a specific form of holistic causality. This suggests the existence of *polymorphous presence*, where the effects of a change or an intervention in one part of a system can be detected in all the other parts of the system, at all its levels. These effects may be of varying weight or import and contrary to one another. We are therefore concerned to pay attention to:

- irreducible emergence – implying levels of reality
- internal relations – implying holistic causality
- laminated systems – implying internal relations between levels of a system
- polymorphous presence – implying internal relations between all elements at all levels of a system.

If critical realism pinpoints the necessity for *integrative pluralism*, what integrates the plurality, i.e. what unifies the specific field of inquiry, preventing an eclectic empiricism of effects? It is not possible to fall back on philosophy, geo-history, political economy, art, literature, the history of Western Civilization, or reconstruction in terms of some grand narrative such as was once provided by e.g. Jean-Jacques Rousseau or Karl Marx. Conceptually concordant heuristics such as "four-planar social being" – i.e. the human being in (a) material transactions with nature; (b) social interactions between agents; (c) social structure proper; and (d) the stratification of the embodied personality, including mental, emotional, and physical being (Bhaskar, 2008b: 160) – can play an important role in relating apparently discrepant but connected fields of inquiry. But it is ultimately only *ex post* and at a relatively late stage in any complex of investigations that we can begin to identify, in a *real definition*, what integrates or unifies the field. That is, it is only at a relatively late stage that we can identify the nature of the specific articulation of the mechanisms in their laminated system. Therefore, in this book, we engage in a double polemic: against both reductionism and eclecticism.

Interdisciplinarity, health, and wellbeing

Nowhere is the need for genuine interdisciplinarity more evident than in research related to health and wellbeing. For a human being is patently a totality and cannot be studied as a congeries of distinct and separable parts. Thus, a person cannot be perceived as being made up of a number of parts that relate to distinct disciplines. (S)he is a totality and therefore requires treatment in a thoroughly interdisciplinary way. The problem is that traditional medicine is dominated by a worldview that is both empiricist, which prevents interdisciplinarity since it omits the non-empirical parts of reality that are necessary for disciplinary integration, and physicalist, which reduces health and wellbeing issues to the biophysical. In order to overcome such barriers, the underlying metatheoretical presuppositions about reality need to be explicit and subject to critical reflection. In short, the rationale for this book on *interdisciplinarity and wellbeing* is that there is a worrying lack of metatheory in discussions on interdisciplinarity. This translates into inadequate health and wellbeing research and ultimately inadequate health practice. As an alternative, we offer a version of health and wellbeing research and practice that we call the "seven enigmas of healing". These enigmas are related to fundamental questions about certain health issues such as: What is it? What are its signs and symptoms? What causes it? All of these enigmas must be re-theorized once the emergence and holistic character of the processes at work are recognized. The seven enigmas offer advice on how to achieve the two functions of contemporary medicine: its *scientific function*, oriented to the understanding of deep (explanatory) causality; and its *healing function*, oriented to the well-functionality of the human being-in-activity in his or her natural and social context. Both require that we understand human beings as a "bio-psycho-social mix" (Sharfstein, 2005).

Fully appreciating the pervasive nature of the real interdisciplinary context radicalizes the practice of health professionals. This is because it implies that a new job or location, or the working through of a fractured relationship with a parent or child, may be the answer to a physical ailment such as a skin complaint, and that a purely physical treatment may need to be complemented by a battery of other measures. For human beings are evolving laminated systems within larger laminated systems. Given our conviction that critical realism is uniquely capable of providing a sound basis for interdisciplinary research, our first aim for this book is to present critical realism. We then elaborate the critical realist implications for interdisciplinarity, which leads to recommendations for researchers, practitioners, and policy-makers.

Outline of the book contents

In Part I of this book, consisting of Chapters 2 and 3, we consider the contradictions – the antinomies – present in contemporary interdisciplinary literature. In Chapter 2, we discuss six features of interdisciplinarity commonly found in the literature, namely: its discussions of the forces driving researchers towards interdisciplinarity; its preoccupation with definitions; its reporting of the failures of interdisciplinarity; its personalistic approach; its comments on the institutional and administrative organization of the interdisciplinary process; and its bibliometric analysis. In Chapter 3 we discuss a seventh characteristic of the interdisciplinarity literature, which is that – in the absence of an adequate metatheoretical justification for interdisciplinarity – researchers characteristically approach interdisciplinary research from the perspective of their particular disciplinary focus.

Part II of this book, which consists of Chapters 4–8, is based on a series of lectures delivered by Roy Bhaskar in 2009 at Örebro University, Sweden. These provide *a general theory of interdisciplinarity from the standpoint of critical realism*. Here we outline the basic concepts of critical realism and consider the theoretical arguments necessary to make applied critical realism (that is, interdisciplinarity) possible. We assume that the relevant object of inquiry is a "laminated system" of a specific type. In Chapter 4, we outline the main concepts of critical realism. However, when we apply basic critical realism to social science, it is necessary to adjust its categories since these were originally developed for the natural sciences. This is done in Chapter 5. In Chapter 6, we develop the basic or core argument for interdisciplinarity. Reference is made to several contexts of interdisciplinarity, such as disability studies, anorexia nervosa, coronary heart disease and HIV education. Starting from the conditions for explanation in open systems, the argument moves through a series of ratchets from multimechanismicity through multidisciplinarity to interdisciplinarity and beyond, developing the notion of a *laminated system*. The basic argument involves a critique of the reductionism and/or atomism which flows from the actualist presuppositions and implications of orthodox philosophy of science. In this way, the argument is oriented against reductionism and atomism in the context of inquiry. However, it is equally oriented against eclecticism in the research cycle, in that it shows how the resultant laminated system can be progressively articulated in the process of science under the influence of empirical, or more generally *a posteriori* (i.e. so as to include qualitative, e.g. hermeneutic), investigations. If the phenomenon of open systems necessitates reference to several distinct mechanisms, of potentially radically different kinds, we indicate the way in which these distinct mechanisms can be intricated in a unitary explanation through the epistemic articulation of the appropriate laminated system, in a real definition of the field of inquiry. In Chapter 7, we focus on the development of critical realism by describing the seven phases of the development of understanding "being". We consider "being" as such, as changing, as whole, as human action, as reflexive, as meaningful, and lastly as unity. In the last chapter of this section, Chapter 8, we further sharpen the characteristics of critical realism by comparing it with other metatheoretical positions and argue that critical realism, in its endeavour to give "the whole picture", embraces the insights of other metatheoretical positions.

In Part III, consisting of Chapters 9–15, we illustrate how interdisciplinarity can be applied in practice. Here, we are interested in the social organization of interdisciplinary research and cooperation. Methodologically speaking, we emphasize integrative pluralism which necessitates a theory of inter-professional cooperation. Specifically, we consider the development of a special theory of interdisciplinarity in health and wellbeing. In Chapter 9, "Biophysical interventions are not enough", we consider those components of health care that are often disregarded because they cannot be reduced to the empirical and/or physical, such as the well-documented placebo effect, which we call the *hidden (holistic) healing ensemble*. In Chapter 10, "The seven enigmas of healing", we refer to certain illnesses/conditions to illustrate the need for the systematic use of interdisciplinarity. In this chapter, the concept of causality moves to the fore, with its complexity in applied/concrete work being stressed. In many ways, this chapter provides the culmination of the thesis so far developed, as we attempt to show how the metatheory of critical realism can be applied in practice. Thus, in the context of each of the *enigmas*, we are faced simultaneously with the spectre of a disjunctive plurality of possible resolutions (e.g. in the case of Enigma 3, diachronically considered, causal aetiologies), each of which is itself composed by another kind of plurality, a conjunctive multiplicity of constituent features or facets (e.g. causes), marking the point of application of interdisciplinarity. Methodological and conceptual sophistication is an important prerequisite to clarity here. We are concerned to relate abstract questions of philosophy to the concrete concerns of healing and care. Thus, the intertwined needs for both a multi- and interdisciplinary approach and a methodologically self-conscious critical realism are brought to the fore. When we integrate our knowledge about mechanisms at different levels into a higher order of knowledge to gain holistic understanding of the totality, the interdisciplinary work becomes itself a new discipline. In principle, this new discipline can be complemented by other disciplines in a new interdisciplinary research programme. For instance, when Darwin came up with his interdisciplinary idea of evolution, this became a new discipline, namely, *evolutionary biology*. This discipline has been complemented by other disciplines, such as genetics, geomorphology, anthropology, and linguistics. In Chapter 11, "The biopsychosocial approach, with special reference to the

International Classification of Functioning, Disability and Health", we analyse and constructively critique the World Health Organization (WHO)'s International Classification of Functioning, Disability and Health (ICF) as a concrete example of how research in health and wellbeing can be approached in an interdisciplinary way. In Chapter 12, "The practical organization of interdisciplinary co-operation", we consider how best to do multi- and interdisciplinary research. While the difference between multidisciplinary and interdisciplinary research is in principle clear, in general the interdisciplinary research project will be conducted by researchers drawn from a multiplicity of disciplines. This raises important questions for the practical implementation of the programmes described in the book. In Chapter 13, "Understanding methodological imperialism", we try to explain the social mechanisms that uphold the problematic but ubiquitous assumption that some methods or methodologies are considered to be "proper" science, while others are considered to be less scientific or even not scientific at all. Specifically, we attempt to understand some of the language-based mechanisms by which methodological imperialism is maintained. In Chapter 14, "Interdisciplinarity in action: explaining the epidemiology of HIV", we illustrate the use of the description, retroduction, elimination, identification, and correction (DREI(C)) dialectic in interdisciplinarity research in a context of HIV education. In the final chapter, Chapter 15, "Concluding considerations", we summarize the main arguments of the book.

The audience of the book

This book will benefit people interested in studying philosophy or the metatheory of interdisciplinarity, and people interested in or seeking to apply critical realism. Therefore, a whole range of applied researchers are likely to find it useful, from advanced undergraduates to postgraduates, to professional researchers in fields such as social work, health, disability research, and indeed any researcher interested in understanding more fully the concrete object of their investigation. However, this book is not only relevant to researchers, but to those people who apply research findings. Therefore, it will prove useful to those concerned with policy and education, such as people in positions of leadership and school and university administrators. In principle this book is relevant to everyone who is interested in doing research into concrete problems or who must professionally apply their skills in the open world of everyday life.

Despite its general appeal, this book is nevertheless intended to be especially valuable for those who are concerned with interdisciplinarity in the field of health and wellbeing. This includes not only professionals such as consultants and researchers, but also commentators, writers, the health media – and of course the patients and the healthy citizens themselves. It is our hope that this book will provide those readers who are not necessarily trained in philosophy with the philosophical ideas and arguments necessary to achieve their interdisciplinary goals.

PART I
Antinomies of mainstream interdisciplinarity

2
OVERVIEW OF THE CONTEMPORARY LITERATURE

There is general agreement in the literature that contemporary approaches to interdisciplinarity are problematic (Siedlok and Hibbert, 2014). For instance, in a survey conducted by the National Academy of Sciences (NAS) (2004: 88), 71% of individual researchers and 90% of provosts reported that "major impediments to interdisciplinarity existed in their institutions". Over the last 50 years, these problems have led to the publication of a large number of books and reports that discuss interdisciplinarity (see e.g. Weingart and Stehr, 2000; Kessel, Rosenfield and Anderson, 2008; Frodeman, 2014). To some extent it is surprising that such problems still exist. This is because the need for interdisciplinarity is well-established, not least because the history of science has excellent examples of the fruitfulness of interdisciplinarity. These include the discovery of DNA, magnetic resonance imaging, the Manhattan Project, laser eye surgery, radar, human genome sequencing, the "green revolution", and manned space flight (NAS, 2004: 17). Interdisciplinarity has also been embraced by many prominent organizations such as the World Health Organization (1986) and European Commission (2014). Therefore, just as there is general agreement that the contemporary practice of interdisciplinarity is problematic, so there is also general agreement that interdisciplinarity is nevertheless highly desirable. However, given the relatively unsuccessful achievement of interdisciplinarity, it seems that the need for interdisciplinarity is unlikely to be satisfied by – is incompatible with – the practice of interdisciplinarity, as it is currently theorized. For this reason, we have entitled this section *Antinomies of Mainstream Interdisciplinarity*. Such antinomies have resulted in certain characteristics of the available academic literature, which we describe later in this chapter. Finally, we also introduce the idea, taken up in more detail later in the book, that many, perhaps all, of these problems can be traced back to an underlying lack of metatheoretical unity.

Most of the literature describes interdisciplinarity, its promises, and its problems in a comprehensive and fairly insightful way. We identified seven distinguishing characteristics of this literature. The first six include: discussions of the forces driving researchers towards interdisciplinarity; a focus on definitions; reporting the problems with interdisciplinarity; a preoccupation with researchers' personal attributes (personalism) as an antidote to the problems of implementing interdisciplinarity; comments on the institutional and administrative organization of the interdisciplinary process; and bibliometric analysis. We also noticed a seventh characteristic which was that – in the absence of a philosophical metatheoretical justification for interdisciplinarity – authors tend to justify interdisciplinarity according to their particular disciplinary focus. Therefore, even when philosophy is not specifically mentioned, there are strands of interdisciplinarity that reflect empiricist (naturalistic) and neo-Kantian and postmodern (anti-naturalistic) philosophical approaches. However, this seventh characteristic of the contemporary interdisciplinarity literature will be explored in Chapter 3.

Driving forces of interdisciplinarity

There are a number of strong forces that drive researchers towards interdisciplinarity. In the report from NAS (2004) four such forces are discussed:

1. the inherent complexity of nature and society;
2. the desire to explore problems and questions that are not confined to a single discipline;
3. the need to solve societal problems, such as environmental problems and active living research; and
4. the power of new technologies.

In respect of the first force, this is an ontological issue that we cannot avoid. As complexity theorists have explained, we live in a complex world and therefore we are going to need interdisciplinarity to understand it (e.g. Gribbin, 2004). A good example of the second force is the development of cognitive science, which includes researchers from, for example, anthropology, neuroscience, linguistics, psychology, and philosophy (e.g. Bermúdez, 2014: 89). We witness the third force in the way that interdisciplinary collaboration is required to deal with the problems associated with tobacco use (e.g. Stokols et al., 2005), or world hunger in the face of climate change (e.g. Vermeulen, Campbell and Ingram, 2012). The internet is a striking example of the fourth force, the power of new technologies.

Defining interdisciplinarity

Many commentators suggest that in order to discuss interdisciplinarity, one has to first give a definition of a discipline (see e.g. Finkenthal, 2001; Moran, 2002). However, this is not a simple assignment since the concept of a discipline is not clear-cut (Becher and Trowler, 2001: 41). Furthermore, other terms have arrived in the literature besides interdisciplinarity, such as cross-, multi-, and transdisciplinarity. Concern with definitions signifies an important attempt to bring clarity to what is at stake, even though it is debatable how fruitful the discussion has been to date. Thus Klein (1990: 56) has emphasized how "terminological hierarchy has played a major role in shaping the way people think about interdisciplinarity". We will provide the critical realist definitions of the various kinds of interdisciplinarity in Chapter 12. However, we will begin by presenting some of the core concepts of critical realism. The critical realist definitions of interdisciplinarity are anchored in ontology, and are not solely derived from epistemology, as are many of the current definitions. We also emphasize the disambiguation of a triple ambiguity in the notion of a "discipline", as follows:

1. between the ontological and epistemological;
2. between the epistemological in the sense of valid knowledge and existing social practice; and
3. between academic research and professional practice.

Interdisciplinarity without metatheory risks failure

A number of interdisciplinary case studies indicate that there is a high risk of failure if metatheoretical issues are not addressed. For example, Sawa (2005) describes how interdisciplinary collaboration collapsed when the involved actors did not share fundamental ontological presumptions. Pohl (2005) shows the complexity of collaboration between natural science researchers and social sciences researchers and their struggle to negotiate different disciplinary "cultures". In an evaluation of transdisciplinary research at the National Institute of Health's Transdisciplinary Tobacco Use Research Centers' programme, Stokols et al. (2005) describe how researchers constituted two different clusters that problematically failed to communicate efficiently, one consisting of neuroscientists and the other consisting of behavioural and social scientists. Such "subgroupings" are rooted in divergent scientific world views. In this book we take the position that a necessary, but not sufficient, condition for successful interdisciplinary scientific collaboration is to explicitly address such metatheoretical issues at the beginning of an interdisciplinary research process.

Preoccupation with personalism

A third characteristic of the literature is the assumption that a major barrier to successful interdisciplinarity is the personality and individual skills of the researchers. Specifically, it looks at how researchers from different fields of knowledge fail to interact and co-operate in order to transcend the boundaries of their own disciplines. In a comprehensive report on interdisciplinary research in the USA (NAS, 2004: 53) it was concluded that "the commonest cause of underperformance of interdisciplinary research is the failure of a team to gel or function collaboratively".

They emphasize how psychological factors are a major reason for this failure to collaborate, such as the tendency for team members to competitively give priority to their individual work. Other commentators, such as Strober (2011), emphasize the problem that researchers from different disciplines use different language and therefore have trouble understanding each other.

However, successful interdisciplinary work is not dependent on personal relations, although they are helpful. For example, the discovery of the helical shape of the DNA molecule was based on the interdisciplinary work of James Watson, Francis Crick, Maurice Wilkins, and Rosalind Franklin. Yet, it would be an exaggeration to say that this quartet constituted a team and collaborated. Sometimes they even refused to talk to each other (Sample, 2010). This example also demonstrates the need for the interdisciplinary process to include shared recognition of the existence of an ontological structure, cognitively appropriated in the epistemological dimension from a number of different vantage points. In other words, the researchers in the DNA example presupposed a common referent, from the perspective of what we call the *intransitive domain* of inquiry. While psychological and shared-language factors may be relevant, it is also necessary to establish a common metatheoretical standpoint, in order for researchers from different disciplines to be "on the same page" so to speak.

Institutional and organizational failings

This brings us to the next important aspect that is highlighted in the literature: the institutionalization and organization of the interdisciplinary process itself. These features include for example funding, institutional homes, publications, and the "division of labour" between the various disciplinary representatives. Such literature points out how the practice of interdisciplinarity is hampered by the following factors: individual disciplines occupy different sections of a university campus; degrees are conferred according to particular disciplines; funding is often skewed towards empiricist or monodisciplinary research; there are few publications willing to publish interdisciplinary research; and career advancement is more difficult for interdisciplinary researchers (NAS, 2004). For instance, the EU's research advisory board (EURAB, 2004) describes the situation as follows:

> The problem is most acute at the fundamental end of the research spectrum, where the traditional one-department, one-discipline structures of most universities are reflected in the structures of the research funding bodies.
> *(Cordis Focus nr 245, 17 May 2004, p. 2)*

Furthermore, EURAB (ibid) address the problems of creating interdisciplinary programmes and issues related to the academic career such as lack of interdisciplinary scientific journals. Clearly, these barriers to interdisciplinarity are significant but in this book we do not discuss all of them at length. We focus on the metatheoretical dimensions of interdisciplinarity. However, some of these barriers will be briefly discussed in Part II where we will show how the basic ideas of the metatheoretical perspective advocated in this book can be organized and applied in interdisciplinary research. We will illustrate our discussion using examples from our experience of interdisciplinary research in disability science (see e.g. Danermark, 2002, 2005; Bhaskar and Danermark, 2006). Nevertheless, it is perhaps important to say at this point a little more about one of these barriers, namely the division of labour between the disciplines. Some critics go so far as to say that we should remove university departments and try to avoid disciplinarity altogether (see Taylor, 2010). To the contrary, we feel that each discipline uses methods that are specific to its subject matter and that acknowledging the usefulness of the different disciplinary approaches is not incommensurable with interdisciplinarity. We think that professional training or certification (such as medical school, law school, architecture school, business school, etc.) can be tremendously useful in ensuring effective practice, although this is not to say that a better understanding of interdisciplinarity within such training would not be helpful.

Bibliometric analysis of interdisciplinary research

The literature frequently contains bibliometric analysis of measures of interdisciplinarity. These measures include: how frequently interdisciplinary research is published; how often researchers quote publications from different disciplinary sources; or the relations between fields of knowledge. Over the last decade, several major national funding bodies have conducted such analyses. This type of quantitative analysis gives information about the clusters of researchers who collaborate. It lists the journals that publish interdisciplinary research and indicates the areas where there is generally a lack of collaboration. On all counts, it reveals that there is a lack of true interdisciplinarity, although there are varying degrees of multidisciplinarity. It has also shown that interdisciplinary research is cited less frequently than monodisciplinary research (see e.g. van Raan, 2000; Morillo, Bordons and Gómez, 2001; Bordons, Morillo and Gómez, 2004; Higher Education Funding Council for England, 2015).

The absence of an adequate metatheoretical perspective

If we take the problems faced by interdisciplinarity as outlined in the literature, and look at them from a critical realist viewpoint, the most striking characteristic is the lack of an adequate metatheoretical perspective. Although we agree with most of the descriptions of the problems of interdisciplinarity – for example, we agree with EURAB that the one-dimensional character of the organization of research is an acute problem – we nevertheless do not agree that these problems exhaust the issue. Instead, we assume that the most basic problem is an insufficiently developed philosophical understanding of the ultimate goal of interdisciplinarity, namely, the integration of knowledge. In this book, we therefore develop an in-depth discussion of *the basic metatheoretical presumptions needed for doing interdisciplinary research*. We

TABLE 2.1 Dimensions, problems, and conditions related to interdisciplinarity

Dimensions	Problems	Conditions
Metatheoretical	No common team philosophy	A common metatheoretical approach
Theoretical	The idea of incommensurability Reductionism	Integration of knowledge Non-reductionism
Methodological	Methodological imperialism	Methods are specific to the level of the analysis (specificity and pluralism in methods)
Individual	Inadequate communication between researchers from different disciplines	Communication is based on mutual understanding of interdisciplinarity and respect for knowledge from other disciplines, education in interdisciplinarity
Administrative	Universities tend to be organized along monodisciplinary lines, lack of career incentives	A supportive administrative structure, clear career pathways for interdisciplinary researchers
Financial/funding	Funding bodies cannot cope with interdisciplinary proposals	Transparent criteria informed by metatheory, equivalent across disciplines, used to evaluate interdisciplinary proposals

therefore underlabour for interdisciplinarity. In Table 2.1, we revisit some of the main problems with interdisciplinarity, as outlined in the literature, and give some examples of how prioritizing the metatheoretical dimension would provide the conditions to avoid such problems.

Although much contemporary interdisciplinarity sidesteps metatheoretical issues altogether, there are instances where metatheory is addressed, but arguably in an inadequate way. In the next chapter, we will discuss these instances, which further reflect the antinomy of the mainstream theory and practice of interdisciplinarity. That is, they reflect contradictions in the way that contemporary researchers from the different disciplines justify or deny the use of interdisciplinary methods.

3
CONTEMPORARY WAYS TO JUSTIFY INTERDISCIPLINARITY

The lack of adequate metatheoretical awareness in discussions of interdisciplinarity results in ambiguity about interdisciplinarity. On the one hand, researchers acknowledge its importance, and on the other hand, they are unclear about how to achieve it (Bammer, 2015). This ambiguity was noted in an ambitious analysis of interdisciplinarity in Sweden, conducted by the Swedish Research Council (Vetenskapsrådet) (2005). In this analysis, the authors reported the existence of competing metatheoretical perspectives on interdisciplinary research, which they called: the pessimistic view; the optimistic view; and the pragmatic view. In the following paragraphs, we expand on their classification.

The pessimistic view

We can discern several arguments against the possibility of interdisciplinarity in the literature. One argument, based in the empiricist, positivistic, quantitative (naturalistic) tradition, claims that – since the only way to obtain reliable knowledge is through statistical generalizations about the way that the world is, and since qualitative studies are case specific and therefore cannot be used to make such generalizations – non-empirical studies are limited in their ability to contribute to broadly applicable knowledge. For instance, Dini, Iqani and Mansell (2011: 3) state, "it is impossible to develop a unified interdisciplinary theoretical framework due to irreconcilable epistemological differences".

Another argument, based in the social construction tradition, takes the truism that mainstream science is inadequately theorized and arrives at the false conclusion that therefore we must give up our belief in ontology and/or that we must accept only local, contextualized truth. As Mackey (1995: 101) states: "there is no place aside from temporal and local context and no truth with a capital T, only the truth within situatedness". For such commentators, "grand" or broadly applicable theories, such as those provided by interdisciplinarity, are questionable. For many of these thinkers, "interdisciplinarity results when different disciplines try to colonize each other" (Balkin, 1996: 952). This position therefore argues that interdisciplinarity has a repressive, imperialist agenda, namely the intention of one discipline to annex the territory of another (Fish, 1989: 19).

The third argument for pessimism takes its point of departure from Thomas Kuhn's idea of paradigms and incommensurability, i.e. that it is not possible to communicate and argue across the borders of a paradigm or problem field. Arguments in one paradigm have no validity in another paradigm. The conclusion is that, since different approaches to science are from different paradigms, therefore they are incommensurable; hence interdisciplinary research is foredoomed to failure (Swedish Research Council (Vetenskapsrådet), 2005: 72).

The optimistic view

There are at least two ways that researchers justify optimism in their approach to interdisciplinarity, based on whether they come from an empiricist or social constructionist/interpretivist viewpoint. If the researchers are empiricists, they can claim to be "interdisciplinary" by:

1. Acknowledging that qualitative research can be used descriptively in the initial (inductive) stages of research, to help researchers to formulate theory and hypotheses (Gilgun, 2001) which can then be tested statistically. This is the view of qualitative research as an important "supporting act" to the main show, namely, empiricist science (Johansson, Risberg and Hamberg, 2003). If statistics are not to be used, the research must be labelled case study research and the researchers must refrain from generalizing the results of the research beyond the boundaries of the research setting (Evera, 1997: 53). Johansson et al. (2003: 10) described this approach as follows: "Qualitative research is valued for its relevance, but is considered lacking in scientific accuracy".
2. Arguing that multiple case studies can be used to make generalizations, and thus be used in broadly applicable interdisciplinary research, but only if they are sufficiently similar. Each case then becomes a sample of the population of similar cases (Krohn, 2010: 38; Evera, 1997: 54).
3. Using non-parametric statistics – if research includes non-numerical (thus qualitative) ranked data, such as expressions of preference (e.g. the number of stars used to rank film quality), this information can be treated statistically in a way that is similar to the way numerical data is treated, with the use of non-parametric statistical analyses. In this way, qualitative data is converted into quantitative data. One could argue that this is interdisciplinary because the difference between qualitative and quantitative data is elided. Also, because it is often researchers in a sociological setting who are likely to use ranked

qualitative data, it would allow such researchers to participate in multidisciplinary research which is dominated by quantitative/empirical scientists, without internal contradiction (Lehmkuhl, 1996).
4. Using research from different natural science disciplines. For example, Burroughs (2007) published an interdisciplinary work on climate change. He reported research from meteorology, geology, geography, biology, and vulcanology. For him, interdisciplinarity meant using research from the perspective of different quantitative disciplines. This optimistic view is anchored in the idea of the unity of the (assumed to be, by definition, empirical) sciences with its roots in the Vienna circle, especially advocated by Otto Neurath [1882–1945], Moritz Schlick [1882–1936], and others. These advocates argue that there is (or should be) a tendency for researchers from different quantitative disciplines to utilize the same methods and that it is in the zones between established disciplines that new knowledge is produced through reconfigurations. Interdisciplinarity in hard systems thinking and complexity theory also tends to fall into this category of optimistic interdisciplinarity. For example, Newell (2001: 1) writes, "The frequent pairing of complexity and interdisciplinarity is no coincidence. It is the contention of this paper that complex systems and phenomena are a necessary condition for interdisciplinary studies".

If the researchers tend towards social constructionism, they will be able to assume equality amongst research paradigms by refusing conceptions of validity or truthfulness altogether – calling them *red herrings* (Newman in Hope and Waterman, 2003) – and reducing empiricist science to just another relativist story amongst research stories (Lather, 1991). If the researchers tend towards the interpretive, they can argue that, if two contexts are similar, then parallels and therefore generalizations can be drawn (remember that it is the accusation that qualitative research is not generalizable that often disqualifies it from being given equal status to empirical research). When this justification for generalization is used, the researchers provide abundant detail about their particular case study, assuming that this detail will encourage readers of the research to find relevant information for their own context. Therefore, interpretive researchers schooled in, for example, the phenomenology of Edmund Husserl [1859–1938] are often encouraged to provide deep, rich, "textured" accounts. The evaluative activity of deciding whether or not there is more-than-local relevance is left up to the reader; it is assumed that this is not the job of the researcher.

The pragmatic view

Some researchers use a certain kind of philosophical pragmatism to permit interdisciplinarity. Many of the currently popular renditions of interdisciplinarity as *transdisciplinarity* – including interdisciplinarity underpinned by the soft systems thinking of e.g. Flood and Jackson (1991) – can be understood in this way. There are also a number of variations of this pragmatic approach to research and truth, and these include:

a   Truth is what a majority think is true, e.g. Lincoln and Guba's (1985) concept of validity as *credibility*. Palmer et al. (2007) demonstrate this pragmatic approach when they use Lincoln and Guba's idea of *member checks* to achieve transdisciplinarity.
b   Truth is the individual's personal truth, e.g. the phenomenologist Sokolowski (2008: 1) makes "the agent of truth" a synonym for "the human person". This approach is used by the transdisciplinary commentator Nicolescu (2006: 142–143), as we see when he states that, "The transcendence inherent in transdisciplinarity is the transcendence of the Subject".
c   Truth is what the marginalized think is true, e.g. the *strong objectivity* of Harding's (2004) *stand-point theory*. Transdisciplinary practitioners Rosendahl et al. (2015) state that, "Transparently assuming positions should not be seen as hindrances, but as an asset. *Strong objectivity* might generate less partial accounts of contested issues" (17; emphasis in original).
d   Truth is what will result in change for the better, e.g. Lather's (1991) *catalytic validity*. Goodley (2010: 23), an interdisciplinary researcher in disability studies, mentions catalytic validity in his argument for foregrounding the political aspects of disabilities.

Another version of the pragmatic view occurs when commentators sidestep the issue of the incommensurability of quantitative and qualitative research, by uncritically assuming the usefulness of each type of research. This version of pragmatism, closely related to point (d), denies the need for metatheory by asking the question "…why should paradigms determine the kind of work one may do with inquiry any more than the amount of illumination should determine where one may conduct a search?" (Howe, 1988: 13). Such a pragmatic approach holds that neither ontology nor epistemology can be placed above practical issues, a view that the pragmatists sometimes call "the dictatorship of the research question" (Tashakkori and Teddlie, 1998: 20).

Some problems with mainstream metatheoretical strategies

We find all of these approaches to interdisciplinarity unsatisfactory. The first perspective, the pessimistic one, is based on a presumption that communication and commensurability are not possible between the different basic schools of thought, an argument that we refute (see Part II, in particular, Chapter 7). In terms of the optimistic and pragmatic approaches, those based on empiricism assume a flat ontology of atomistic events and therefore it is questionable that they are indeed interdisciplinary as they remain reductionist. Those approaches based on interpretivism or social constructionism tend to be irrealist and relativist, amongst other things. Flood and Jackson (1991), whose approach to systems theory is often used as a metatheoretical approach to interdisciplinarity, reveal their irrealism when they state that, "In the modern systems approach, the concept *system* is used not to refer to things in the world but to a particular way of organising our thoughts about the world" (2; emphasis in original). Nowotny (2004: 11) provides a good example of relativism when she writes:

> Quality control is indeed a very tricky criterion. In our first book, we readily admitted ... that this is transdisciplinarity's Achilles' heel. ... There is no single criterion as there is in disciplinary quality control, where one can always fall back on the standards used in the discipline, allowing one to say: this is good physics, good biology, or good geology. You don't have this anymore.

Problematically, but nevertheless usefully because it reduces professional conflict, both empiricists and interpretivists/social constructionists agree on two things. First, they agree that interdisciplinary research should avoid offering universally relevant, ontologically deep causal mechanisms (theories) to explain phenomena: the former because they have a shallow, constant-conjunction understanding of causality; the latter because they celebrate particularism and see no possibility of arriving at universal, grand theories. The consequence is that, whether researchers are quantitatively or qualitatively orientated, their interdisciplinary research results in eclecticism – described by Turner (1990: 1) as "a fragmentary pastiche of disciplines" – rather than intellectual integration. Second, and also unlike the critical realist position, both the empiricists and the interpretivists/social constructionists agree that there is an irreconcilable dichotomy between facts and values. Therefore, empiricist science cannot inform human values. For the empiricists, this simply means that they must be careful to avoid values, leaving them up to the non-empiricists (Rittel and Webber, 1973). For the practitioners of interpretive/social constructionist approaches, this means that they may explore values but these values are forever divorced from facts. Thus, values, in typical Kantian style, are assumed to exist in a different realm of (split) reality, associated with a transcendent subject (Nicolescu, 2006; Max-Neef, 2005). Since we use values to decide action, the fact/value dichotomy is devastating for rational action and it results in a contradiction between the common-sense or lay understanding of science – that it provides guidance for action and policy decisions (action in wider society) – and the philosophical understanding of science. This contradiction can be exploited by unscrupulous policy-makers, who, when it suits them, can use the contemporary philosophical understanding of the function of science to disregard factually-based action imperatives using the argument that the individual – the transcendent subject – must decide his/her own values. Thus, facts supposedly do not inform individual or social values. However, if the facts indicate an action that suits the policy-makers, they can use the common-sense or lay understanding of the function of science to justify using these facts to guide social policy to ensure the action.

Suffice to say that in this book we propose an alternative perspective that will resolve these antinomies. In Part I of this book, we hinted at the challenges facing interdisciplinary researchers. We now move to Part II, in which we provide an outline of the philosophy of critical realism. Our aim is to provide the reader with important conceptual tools in support of our main argument which is that, due to the complexity of issues related to health and wellbeing, there is an urgent need for an adequate theory of interdisciplinarity.

PART II
A critical realist general theory of interdisciplinarity

4

CORE CONCEPTS OF CRITICAL REALISM

This chapter is an abridged overview of critical realism. However, many of the ideas introduced here will be revisited and deepened in subsequent chapters. We begin with a discussion of five features of critical realist philosophy, specifically: its conception of the role of philosophy; its characteristic of *seriousness*; its understanding of the nature of philosophical argument; its understanding of the nature of philosophy itself; and its idea of *enhanced reflexivity*. We also explore the critical realist idea that reality is stratified and that science is about discovering the nature of things not immediately apparent or obvious to our everyday experience. As such, critical realism allows a hopeful vision of science; it is something that we can use to create positive change in our world.

The role of philosophy

Critical realism is an underlabourer for the various sciences and practices. The person who initiated this metaphor, John Locke (1979/1689: 9–10), said:

> The Commonwealth of Learning is not at this time without Master-Builders, whose mighty designs, in advancing the Sciences, will leave lasting monuments to the Admiration of Posterity. But everyone must not hope to be a Boyle, or a Sydenham; and in an Age that produces such Masters, as the Great Huygenius, and the Incomparable Mr. Newton, and some others of that strain; 'tis ambition enough to be employed as an under labourer in clearing the ground a little, and removing some of the rubbish that lies in the way to knowledge.

This is what critical realism attempts to do, and in so doing, we come to the second point.

Seriousness

Critical realism adopts the standpoint of seriousness. This derives from Georg Wilhelm Friedrich Hegel [1770–1831] who was critical of the assumptions of Kantian and empiricist philosophy, which he felt had little practical relevance to the pressing issues of his time. An example of this un-seriousness in much contemporary philosophy is found in the work of David Hume [1711–1776], the British empiricist. Hume (2008/1779, Part I) remarked that there are no better grounds for going out of a room by the ground-floor exit than by the second-floor window. This is not a serious proposition; because if Hume were being serious then he ought to leave by the second-floor window at least 50 per cent of the time. However, he always left by the ground-floor exit, and for good reason; if he left from the second-floor window, the force of gravity would pull him to the ground and he might break a leg or worse. So Hume's position was not serious in the sense that his position is not applicable in the context of everyday life. Another suggestion from Hume (1934/1740, Book II, Section III) that indicates a lack of seriousness in ethical affairs is that there is no reason to prefer the scratching of one's little finger to the destruction of the whole world. But this is an odd position, for if it were true then you could never argue for anything in moral affairs; you could not establish that it is better to sacrifice your little finger and save the world. Of course, what is wrong here is that if the world goes, then you lose your little finger as well. Essentially, to achieve this statement, it is necessary for Hume to detotalize himself; that is, he must take himself out of the practical totality that includes the rest of the world. This is a characteristic feature of much academic philosophy, since it hypostatizes or abstracts itself from the rest of the world. Critical realism, by contrast, produces philosophy that is of practical relevance to our everyday lives.

The nature of philosophical argument

The third feature of critical realism is its conception of the nature of philosophical argument. According to critical realism, philosophical argument always takes the form of immanent critique. This means that you do not start a philosophical argument from your own premises. Rather you take the premises of your discussant, that is, the person that you are discussing something with or whose opinion you want to contest. You then show that, when properly considered, these premises entail a conclusion that your discussant would find objectionable. What you are doing is always referring to, and starting from, someone else's premises, not your own. A little reflection will show that this is the only way that you can ever conduct a convincing argument with someone else. You have to talk to them about something that is relevant to their own belief system. This is the critical realist method of immanent critique.

The nature of philosophy itself

The fourth feature of critical realist philosophy is its assumption about the nature of philosophy itself. According to critical realism, philosophy does not consider a realm apart from that of scientific practices, or everyday experience and presuppositions. It is not concerned with some ideal world of Platonic forms or something of that sort. Critical realism considers just exactly this world here, but from the standpoint of what scientific or ordinary activity or discourse presupposes about it. If you are asked, for example, how many people are in a room, you would probably count the number of heads and come to a figure, say 45. However, if someone in the room is speaking on their mobile phone to someone else, then there is also a sense in which the person at the end of the phone line could be in the room. You would then have to ask why the head count is necessary. If the context is a lecture, and the head count is for the purposes of how many cups to lay out for tea, then the person present via the phone would not be counted. However, if the purpose is to provide course handouts, and the person on the phone is a part of the course but on this occasion is absent, then they should be counted so that their friend can pass the handouts to them later. Thus it is important to see that "the number of people in this room" is ambiguous. The ambiguity would be further highlighted if we tried to count how many *things* are present in a room, because what counts as a *thing*? The point of philosophy is therefore to bring out what is involved in our discourse about some subject matter by looking at its presuppositions. So just to repeat, philosophy is about this world, this one world, but from the point of view of its most abstract qualities. All of these features of philosophy help us to arrive at greater reflexivity and this brings us to the fifth feature of critical realist philosophy, specifically, enhanced reflexivity.

Enhanced reflexivity

Reflexivity in its most basic form specifies the capacity of an agent or an institution to monitor and account for its activity. Critical realism is primarily concerned to enhance our reflexivity, that is, to give a better account (theory) of what it is that we do in the world (practice). Although the critical realist philosophy of science is critical of theories about what scientists do, this is a means to an end. Ultimately, critical realism is more concerned with the way that, in the social domain or perhaps even in natural sciences with social implications, the function of science is to be substantially critical of some of the practices in which we engage. In this way, critical realist philosophy has a transformative and potentially emancipatory role.

These five features – underlabouring, seriousness, immanent critique, the conception of philosophy as explicating presuppositions of human activities, and enhanced reflexivity in the social field – potentially transform practice. They are designed to produce a philosophy that is practical and relevant. You can therefore use critical realism to make better sense of what is happening in the house in which you live or to explain some puzzling or important event that is happening in the world.

Critical realism and ontology

At one time, the whole idea of ontology, of realism, or of the necessity of the practical relevance of philosophy, was to a certain extent taboo. Roy Bhaskar started his PhD studies doing a thesis on the relevance of economic theory for underdeveloped countries. However, at the time – in the 1970s when neoclassical economics was dominant – it was accepted that economists should never discuss the relevance of their economic doctrine or metatheory to the world. Instead, it was assumed that the job of economic scholars was to show how many deductive implications could be derived from a set of assumptions. According to Friedman [1912–2006] and the other methodologists at the time, one was not allowed to ask whether these assumptions were realistic or not. Therefore, Bhaskar was soon forced to realize that he could not continue with his PhD because he was not allowed to say anything about the relevance of economic theory for underdeveloped countries. This motivated him to explore the philosophy of science and ultimately philosophy. In terms of the philosophy of science, Bhaskar was shocked to discover that everything discussed concerned epistemology or things to do with our knowledge of the world; there was no actual discussion of the world. Therefore, the philosophy of science was confined to discussions about confirmation or falsification theory, elaboration, explanation, or prediction – conceived as processes that take place within knowledge. Intuitively, Bhaskar thought that there was something very wrong going on. To find out what this might be, he went further back into philosophy and ultimately discovered the problem; clearly stated by Kant and Hume was the assertion that you cannot "do" ontology. Just to clarify, ontology is traditionally regarded as being the study of the world and it is counterpoised to epistemology which is traditionally regarded as the study of knowledge. However, Kant and Hume declared an embargo on ontology. This deep-rooted assumption within the modern analytical tradition infects both of its main wings, which are empiricism and neo-Kantianism. We will also discuss other positions such as social constructivism and hermeneutics later in this book.

A new ontology

Bhaskar realized that a strong argument was needed to re-establish the legitimacy of asking ontological questions about the world. However, it seemed to him that this argument for ontology (reality) would have to be supplemented by another argument. This was because, although contemporary scientists and philosophers theoretically deny the existence of ontology, their statements nevertheless tacitly assume an ontology, and their actions belie their theoretical denial of ontology. However, the kind of ontology presupposed by the actions of scientists is problematic. To illustrate this, take Hume's doctrine that a causal law is a constant conjunction of atomistic events. It implies an ontology in which reality repeats itself since, whenever there is one empirical feature, this is always correlated with another empirical feature. Furthermore, it implies that the world is flat, i.e. is made up only of empirical entities, irrespective of the domain of reality in question. Hume's empiricism also presupposes that the world is unchanging. However, contrary to this position, it seemed intuitively obvious to Bhaskar that the world is structured, differentiated, and changing. Bhaskar therefore took on the following tasks: (a) to show how all philosophy and discourse presupposes ontology, even if it contradictorily also denies that ontology; (b) to explain why the implicitly presupposed Humean ontology of a flat, undifferentiated, unchanging world is wrong; and (c) to establish in its place a new ontology. The original brief of critical realism was therefore as follows: to establish the legitimacy of ontology; and to establish the nature of a new ontology.

An immanent critique of Humean ontology

According to the critical realist presupposition mentioned previously, to achieve his objective, Bhaskar needed to carry out an immanent critique. He could not simply claim that, from his point of view, the world is structured, differentiated, and changing. This would have held little water because it would simply have set his beliefs against those implicit in empiricism and neo-Kantianism. Instead he had to focus on a feature in existing philosophy that he could show was inconsistent with the assumption of a flat, undifferentiated, and unchanging world. The feature that he chose was the experimental activity of scientists. This was because, despite their disagreements about the nature of science, philosophers, at least in the West, are committed to the idea that experimentation is an important feature of it. Bhaskar therefore undertook a transcendental analysis of science. *Transcendental* simply means that Bhaskar undertook an analysis of science from the standpoint of its most basic presuppositions. In this case he asked: What is it about the nature of the world that experimentation presupposes?

When scientists set up an experiment, they artificially isolate a bit of reality in order to produce a result that otherwise would not be forthcoming. This activity allows them to have access to the workings of mechanisms that are registered in statements of law. This activity is only significant on the basis of the assumption that the laws that they identify continue to operate outside the closed system set up by the experimental scientist. In other words, we assume that the law of gravity operates on us in ordinary life outside the laboratory conditions under which we might test it. The force of gravity is operating on a stationary seated person in exactly the same way that it would if they, or Hume, were hurtling out of the second-floor window, falling down to the ground. It just so happens that in the open system in which we live, gravity is counteracted by other tendencies and forces. This fundamental assumption of the experimental method – namely that the mechanisms and structures identified under experimental conditions continue to operate outside the experimental context, combined with the open-system nature of the world – means there are no constant conjunctions of events outside the experimental context. It is thus established that laws – and the workings of mechanisms and structures generally – cannot be the same as constant conjunctions of events. *Even when there are no constant conjunctions of events*, mechanisms and structures continue to operate. Laws are therefore "transfactual"; and the idea of the transfactuality of laws fatally undermines the idea of Humean ontology and its assumption that constant conjunctions are the only way to know causality.

This argument does two things. First, it produces an argument for ontology, because it is a statement about the world. Specifically, it is a statement about how the world must be for experimentally produced knowledge to be possible (amongst other things). Second, it produces an argument for a characteristically new ontology because it claims that there is a profound disjuncture or mismatch between, on the one hand, generative mechanisms and structures and scientific laws, and on the other hand, patterns of events identified in experience. Accordingly – and contrary to empiricist and neo-Kantian accounts – reality has a depth to it. This argument is useful in helping us to achieve the two objectives of critical realism: the objective that we want to be able to say something about the world, i.e. that we want to be able to "do" a philosophical ontology; and the objective that we want a new ontology, i.e. an ontology that will be true to the fundamental features of the world.

In terms of the first objective, this argument suggests a critique of the *epistemic fallacy*, that is, the reduction of being to knowledge, or the reduction of ontological to epistemological questions. The epistemic fallacy is the assumption that you can always analyse "being" in terms of "our knowledge of being". To counter the epistemic fallacy, Bhaskar suggests that there are two dimensions to science: the *transitive* and *intransitive* dimensions. The transitive dimension is that aspect of knowledge that involves people and their beliefs, or scientists and their theories. From the point of view of the transitive dimension, the scientist's work proceeds by the critique and transformation of pre-existing social products. Science is therefore a commodity, and like other commodities, it is part of the social world. However, we also have a world which exists independently of people and their beliefs and this is the intransitive dimension.

The epistemic fallacy is the idea that pre-existing philosophy attempts to analyse the world (i.e. being or statements about being) in terms of knowledge (i.e. statements about knowledge). An example of the prevalence of this kind of assumption in pre-existing philosophy is provided by Wittgenstein (1999/1922: 102) who wrote: "Laws, like the law of causation, etc., treat of the network and not of what the network describes". For Wittgenstein it was therefore sufficient only to analyse the network; he argued that we do not need to explore what the network describes. Critical realists agree that there is a network, but that (a) it is a complicated social network and therefore we must understand its laws and rhythms; and (b) there are things that exist outside the network. It is therefore possible to be both an ontological realist, that is, one can believe that the real world exists and that it has certain deep features, and an epistemological relativist, that is, one can believe that all knowledge is socially produced and is transient, or fallible. Therefore, all knowledge will be replaced or sublimated in time; there is no opposition or contradiction between relativism, conceived as epistemological, and realism, conceived as ontological. The third thing implied by ontological realism and epistemological relativism is that, although all beliefs are socially produced and therefore socially changing, we do have objective grounds – which can be specified in a particular domain – for preferring one belief over another, called *judgemental rationality*. For example, theory A can be judged as preferable to theory B, in virtue of its ability to explain not only those aspects of reality explained by theory B, but also some additional features. Consider the competing theories of Newton and Einstein. If we describe the world using Newton's theory and it explains n features of reality, and then we describe the world using Einstein's theory and it explains n + 9 features of reality, it is valid to prefer the n + 9 option. These three things, namely ontological realism, epistemological relativism, and judgemental rationality, are key ideas underlying critical realism.

The domains of the real, the actual, and the empirical

It is only possible to make sense of experimental activity if one assumes that the structures and mechanisms identified *inside* the laboratory nevertheless continue to exist and act *outside* the laboratory. This means that real structures and mechanisms cannot be reduced to actual patterns of events and constant conjunctions as measured inside the laboratory. Therefore, one has to differentiate between the domain of the real and the domain of the actual. However, not all that is actual can be experienced, which leads to the idea that there are three domains: the domain of the real, the domain of the actual, and the domain of the empirical. Not all of the real is actual; and not all of the actual is empirical. Therefore, it is possible to have structures and causal laws existing unactualized and independently of a particular pattern of events. It is also possible to have patterns of events existing independently of their experience.

The dialectic of science

From this standpoint, science is essentially the move from patterns of events to structures. In other words, science is a continual unearthing of new structures and mechanisms. This makes science exciting and recondite with respect to ordinary experience. Science is therefore about discovering the nature of things not immediately apparent or obvious to common sense and our everyday experience. It is about uncovering fundamental causal mechanisms and generative structures that happen, speaking metaphorically, behind the revealed pattern of events. Furthermore, the nature of the world is not only stratified but in principle this stratification is multi-tiered. For example, a table is constituted by molecules, the molecules are constituted by atoms, the atoms are constituted by electrons, and the electrons in turn are constituted by quarks or the quantum field. We therefore have five levels of structure which science has identified in the material world. However, the stratification of science is in principle unending. What happens in the case of any particular science is an epistemological dialectic which will take you from one level of stratified reality to another. This is the logic of scientific discovery. One starts at one level, with a description of that level of reality. The next step is to think of plausible mechanisms that explain why reality is the way that it is perceived to be. This step is called retroduction. Thus, *description* is the first moment, and *retroduction* is the second moment. However, at the second moment one will in principle have a plurality of possible theories. It is therefore necessary to choose between them and this takes us to the third step in the scientific dialectic, namely *elimination*. Here we ask whether our theory offers the best explanation of the available evidence compared to rival theories. Ultimately one will arrive at the fourth level, which is *identification*. At the stage of identification, it may (or may not) be possible to refine one's perceptual instruments to observe the structure or mechanism and to carry out experiments and test hypotheses in closed-system laboratory-style contexts. However, sometimes the structure or mechanism can only be detected through its effects (i.e. it cannot be directly measured). We can nevertheless "test" our theory by checking that it explains even small characteristics of the issue at hand, by evaluating interventions suggested by the knowledge (do they result in expected outcomes, and if not, is this explainable due to open-system mediations or is there a problem with our theory?), and by looking for other instances where our theory might apply, to ascertain whether it can explain these instances too. At this (usually) inter-subjective fourth level, a new level of reality has been described. It is now possible to begin a new round of the scientific dialectic. Therefore, at this new second level of reality, one can retroduct the generative mechanism responsible for it, leading to a plurality of possible explanations, the best of which is chosen through elimination, followed by identification, and so on. Nevertheless, during the process of identification, it may become necessary to refine the concepts of the previous levels. This suggests a fifth stage in the dialectic of science, namely *correction* of all the previous stages. Therefore, the dialectic of science can be summarized as: description, retroduction, elimination, identification, and correction, also known as the DREI(C). In Chapter 5, we will describe critical realism's further development of this basic form of the logic of scientific discovery when highlighting the differences in natural sciences and social sciences and their implications for the logic.

Three senses in which reality is structured

Up to this point, we have isolated two senses in which critical realism describes reality as being structured. First, there is a sense in which you need a distinction between the real and the actual. The necessity for this sense is the existence of real structures and mechanisms that are irreducible to the actual patterns of events. Second, there is the sense in which reality has a multi-tiered stratification. Therefore, tables are composed of molecules, which are composed of atoms, which are generated or composed of such things as electrons. However, critical realism suggests a third fundamental kind of stratification, or inflection to the idea of stratification, which is *emergence*. Examples of an emergent level of reality include the way that the level of mind emerges from the level of the body, or the way that the level of society emerges from the level of human beings. When you have an emergent level of reality, you have three implied conditions. The first is that the higher-order or emergent level is unilaterally dependent on the lower-order level. In other words, you have mind dependent on body but you don't have body dependent on mind. Second, you have taxonomic irreducibility, for example, there is no way in which you can understand the intentional behaviour of human beings solely by reference to physical features. You have to understand intentional behaviour by reference to things like motives and rules, and reasons and so forth. You cannot understand it by reference to the properties of the lower-order levels. The third feature is not just taxonomic irreducibility but causal irreducibility. Causal irreducibility means that the state of the higher-order level provides the causally efficacious conditions for the state of the lower-order level. For example, you might ask someone to get you some coffee. If the person says yes, your speech action will have initiated a sequence of events that will ultimately result in the coffee being placed into your hands. This is the kind of effect that human beings are having on the environment, such as global warming, and it is a necessary condition for any intentional action. The point of this book is to help readers to see the world in a different way, leading them to do different things. Furthermore, the readers will be doing different things physically, because mind is unilaterally dependent on body and so the physical states of the world will be different as a result of our intentional action to write this book. If we are hungry and we need a meal or a break, the assumption is that a coffee break will provide a means for us to refresh and replenish our physical metabolism. Therefore, in a way, this offers hope for change because the way that human beings act in the world is continuous with the way that we are emergent entities in the world, and thus are able to produce effects within it.

In this chapter, we have considered five features of critical realism designed to make it a practical philosophy, not only from the point of view of research, but from the point of view of everyday life. We have therefore looked at: philosophical underlabouring; the idea of "seriousness", or the unity of theory and practice; the need for internal or immanent critique; the conception of philosophy as explicating presuppositions of human activities; and the conception of the role of critical realism in a discipline or field as promoting enhanced reflexivity and/or transformed practice. We have also looked at two fundamental theorems within critical realism. The first turns on the critique of the epistemic fallacy, i.e. the irreducibility of ontology to epistemology and leads to the conception that there are two domains of science: the transitive and the intransitive. The second turns on the critique of actualism, which is the idea that reality merely consists of actualities or patterns of events, and that there are no structures or causal machinery to explain how these events happen. It leads to the critical realist idea that the world is structured and that the aim of science is to discover the structures and mechanisms that make things happen. This process is in principle infinite within any one branch of science; we therefore have a multi-tiered stratification of reality. Finally, we looked at three conditions for emergent structures or levels: unilateral dependence, taxonomic irreducibility, and causal irreducibility. We now turn to how critical realism can help us to improve the way that we carry out social science.

5

CRITICAL REALISM AND SOCIAL SCIENCE

This chapter considers how the categories of basic critical realism, originally designed for the natural sciences, must be adjusted to address social science issues. While metatheoretical unity is necessary for interdisciplinarity – in some key ways science is the same for both the natural and the social sciences – this unity does not require that we deal with the subject matter of the natural sciences in the same way that we deal with the subject matter of the social sciences. To fail to adjust basic critical realism for use in the social sciences would be to mistakenly assume that the social sciences are a deductive elaboration or instantiation of the natural sciences. This would be the opposite of the underlabourer conception of science. Instead it is necessary to undertake an independent analysis of social science and to look at the conditions of the possibility of social science. Because of this analysis, it may become apparent that some features of the social sciences are the same as for the natural sciences. This chapter is therefore about the modifications that we need to make to original critical realism when we are dealing with the social world. It provides a generalized social ontology and outlines its implications for interdisciplinary social research, and public health policy and planning.

In Chapter 4, we provided the critical realist argument for a new ontology. This argument establishes that the world is structured and differentiated and that there is a radical difference between: (a) generative mechanisms and causal structures, (b) patterns of events, and (c) empirical regularities. This central, initial argument of critical realism can be developed in various ways. One way, which we look at in this chapter, is to ask: Can you apply the conceptual apparatus (theories) of generative mechanisms and causal structures to social life, and if so, how do we test these social theories? Do they have distinctive features that they do not share with natural scientific theories?

These questions were answered by Bhaskar (2014/1979) in his second book: *The Possibility of Naturalism*. At the time that this book was written, there were certain dichotomies and dualisms which were characteristic of the social sciences, social theory, and philosophy of social science. These dualisms included:

1. structure and agency;
2. individualism and collectivism, that is, the individual and the whole or the collective;
3. naturalistic and anti-naturalistic approaches, such as positivism and hermeneutics, that is, meaning and law.

We often find these dualisms in the thinking and discussions that researchers have about their work. For example, researchers often wonder whether they should investigate social scientific subject matters by (a) seeking the meaning that agents place on what they do or the meaning that they have in society, or (b) investigating empirical, law-like behaviour, empirical regularities – eventually formulating social scientific laws which will be analogous to natural scientific laws like the law of gravity. This is the dualistic dispute between positivism and hermeneutics, or more generally between naturalism and anti-naturalism. These are the three major macro dichotomies, but there are also micro dichotomies in the human sciences. For example, there are the micro dichotomies between mind and body, reason and cause, fact and value, and theory and practice. The claim of *The Possibility of Naturalism* is that these dichotomies can be rationally resolved on the basis of a better and more adequate account of social science (or social and psychological science).

Structure and agency

Let us take the dualism between structure and agency. This dualism is classically represented by the contrast between followers of two important sociologists: Emil Durkheim [1858–1917], who stressed structure; and Max Weber [1864–1920], who stressed agency. This dualism can also be understood in terms of the arguments from Chapter 4. Basically we are asking: Are there structures at work in social life analogous to the generative mechanisms of nature and, if so, what are they? Thinking of the problem in terms of structure and agency, it is self-evident that society pre-exists us, individual human beings; nevertheless, it does not exist independently of the activity of human beings. Therefore, society pre-exists, but is reproduced or transformed by, human beings. This analysis means that a temporal dimension is very important for social science because, for any individual or any generation or any moment of time or any cohort, there are certain things that pre-exist them. These pre-existing things will include the structures and everything else that is considered part of society. The agent makes use of what pre-exists to carry out their particular acts and, as a result of their action, the social structure and the rest of society will be reproduced or transformed. It is crucial to note that, in this process, structure and agency will be different. For example, the reason that you might want to get married to someone is not to reproduce the rules and conventions of marriage. When you buy commodities at a shop, it is not to reproduce capitalism or to reproduce the monetary or banking systems. Reproducing the institution of marriage, capitalism, or the monetary system is the unintended product or consequence of one's actions. One therefore must think in terms of two levels: a level of agency and a level of structure. The social structure is what the agent makes use of in carrying out their acts. In virtue of their activity, and the activity of other agents, the social structure is reproduced or transformed. Time is also important in this process: some social form or social structure exists at a period T1; and then an agent carries out an action at period T2; and as a result at period T3 the social structure or other social forms are reproduced or transformed. Critical realists call this the Transformational Model of Social Activity (TMSA).

The TMSA is similar to Anthony Giddens' (1986) Structuration Theory, because both agree that you do not have structure without agency and you do not have agency without structure. These two aspects of social life mutually implicate each other. However, unlike Structuration Theory, the TMSA suggests that structure pre-exists agency; and as such it is always a constraint on agency. The problem with Structuration Theory is that it suggests that when we go to sleep in a society, society itself also goes to sleep. When we wake up in the morning, we can therefore create another society. Unfortunately, social transformation is much more difficult than this. Both Bhaskar and Giddens initially thought that the TMSA was essentially the same as Structuration Theory; it was Bhaskar's colleague, Margaret Archer, who pointed out they were different and that the main difference was that Structuration Theory lacked the component of time.

Later Bhaskar (2008b/1993: 160) elaborated the TMSA into the model of Four-Planar Social Being, based on the idea that social life is not just a matter of agency and structure; it also takes place in nature (Figure 5.1). Furthermore, it involves two aspects, at the very least, of activity since the agents themselves have a profound stratification. The model of Four-Planar Social Being is therefore a critical realist elaboration and resolution of the dualism between structure and agency. It consists of four dimensions:

1. material transactions with nature;
2. social interactions between people;
3. social structure per se (such as economic structures); and
4. the stratification of the embodied personality.

The individual and the collective

Let us look at what critical realism says about the relationship between the individual and the collective. Methodological individualists such as Karl Popper [1902–1994] assumed that anything that was not individualist would have to be magically summoned forth as the behaviour of masses of individuals. However, this is to misconstrue the non-individualist approach to social science, because in sociology and social sciences we are not concerned about the behaviour of masses of individuals. Rather we are concerned about the behaviour of the persistent relations

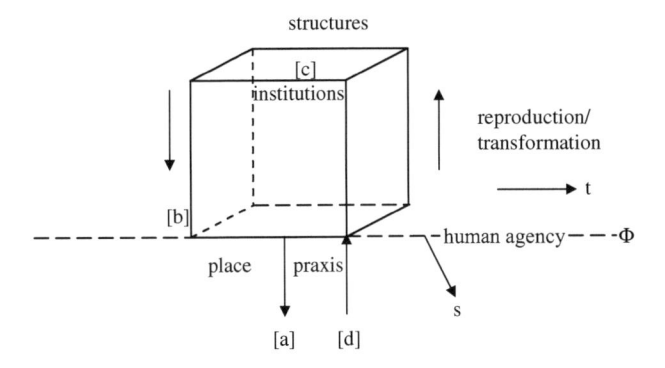

FIGURE 5.1 Social life and wellbeing in the context of four-planar social being
Source: Bhaskar (2008b/1993: 160).

between individuals. These are enduring relations: such as those between the citizen and the member of parliament; between the capitalist and the worker; between the bank manager and the person or firm who gets credit; between husband and wife; or between parents and children.

However, another way to look at social life is in terms of orders of scale. In principle, a researcher can invent any order of scale to suit their purpose, but here we will suggest seven orders or laminations of scale that may be relevant in social science (Bhaskar, 2010: 9–10):

1. The first level of scale is the sub-individual, looking at things like the unconscious, the preconscious, or motives, drives, desires, aspirations, hopes, dreams, and fantasies of a particular individual. This is the world of Freud [1856–1939], Jung [1875–1961], and psychologists.
2. The second level of scale is the individual and this is the level at which we might want to write the biography of an individual. This is the level which fascinated Sartre [1905–1980]; his intellectual career ended in trying to write the biography of Stalin. He thought that this was ultimately how one should carry out social science. Critical realists agree that it is important to understand individual biographies in social science, but it is also important to look at what happened in the Soviet Union in terms of these other dimensions of scale.
3. The third level of scale is the micro-social and this is the level of Erving Goffman [1922–1982] and Harold Garfinkel [1917–2011]. This is the level at which we might analyse things like turn-taking in telephone conversations, or how it is that we do not bump into each other while walking on pavements.
4. The fourth level is the level of classical sociology. This is the structural level, at which we might want to think of, for instance, the relations between capitalists and workers; or how a person with suicidal tendencies relates to work (see Durkheim, 2005/1897). This fourth level is the middle social level.
5. The fifth macro level of scale is where we might want to investigate properties or features of society as a whole, for instance the French educational system

might be a topic of interest (see Archer and Vaughan, 1971). And of course France is itself in a larger context, and therefore this leads to the next level.
6. The sixth level of scale is where we might want to take into account the geo-historical trajectory of something like Christianity, colonialism, or capitalism.
7. The seventh level of scale would be the world as a whole. An example of an academic who has been working at this level is Wallerstein (1992), who developed world-systems theory (also known as world-systems analysis or the world-systems perspective).

Like most of the categorizations within critical realism, it is important not to think of these domains, strata, or levels as a hierarchy; we do not want to prioritize them. In principle, any level either above or below the level that one is investigating may be involved in the explanation. Critical realists emphasize that relations do not only work in one direction; therefore, it is not just a case of human beings having causal effects on nature per se, but nature also has causal effects on the other levels. Therefore, there is an interaction between these different levels and in principle this interaction travels both upwards and downwards.

Meaning and law

The third dichotomy that critical realists are critical of is the dichotomy between meaning and law. It is important to understand that human beings are radically different from natural things. In particular they have reasons for doing what they do. They act intentionally; and this means that individual human beings have a subjective side that one does not find in nature. Furthermore, there are rules and belief systems (social forms) that are themselves part of the subject matter of social science. This is what the hermeneuticists, the anti-naturalists, have always stressed. Typically, however, they moved from this true premise to the false conclusion, based on positivism, that therefore the social sciences or social studies must pursue a radically different method from the natural sciences. For example, the English philosopher Peter Winch [1926–1997] says that because social life has an intelligibility that the natural world does not have, we cannot use the same methods for social science that we use for natural science. In one way, we completely agree with him. It is true that the social world does have an intelligibility and that the intelligibility of the social world is in part composed of the reasons that people have for doing what they are doing. However, the natural world is also intelligible and there are mechanisms that explain why things happen in both the natural and social worlds.

The second argument for the dichotomy between meaning and law is that there is no physical existence in society apart from bodies. However, there are many natural objects of investigation that have no physical existence. Gravity is not something that physically exists. A magnetic field is also not something that physically exists; rather it is something which produces effects on physical, material things. The whole argument can be slightly pedantic; and an important point must be conceded to hermeneuticists, which is that there are certain properties possessed by human beings and societies that natural objects do not possess. This critical realism totally accepts. However, while social forms and human actions have an irreducible conceptual aspect, this does not exhaust them. If we take as an example something like war, perhaps it is true that a necessary condition to having a war is that we have a concept of a war. However, when we change the concept, it does not mean that we have peace. War is something more than having a concept; it is fighting and it is brutish in the same way that hunger and poverty are something more than their concepts. Therefore, critical realism argues that hermeneutics defines the starting point of social science. It gives us our datum. It is what we start with, that is, we start with the reasons that the agents will give for the things that they do. But it does not end there. Indeed, in principle, we can critique the conceptions held by the agents, that is, we may regard the agents themselves as corrigible. For example, such corrigibility is demonstrated in cases of Freudian rationalization. Education or research is a process whereby one gains deeper interpretations, understandings, or conceptions of the natural and the social worlds; and this implies that some interpretations are too simple or even incorrect.

In other words, the hermeneuticists have correctly isolated the real difference between the natural and social sciences, namely the conceptual character of social life. Critical realism adds that it is at this exact point – the conceptual character of social life – that we must start our social research. That is, social research must necessarily begin at the point of agents' conceptions. However, hermeneutics is not the end of the matter as, in some cases, non-hermeneutical procedures may also be necessary. For instance, it may be important to your study that you count the number of suicides, or calculate the number of cases of drug abuse. Therefore, statistics also have a role in social research. Furthermore, in the process of deepening your understanding of the subject matter, you may eventually reach a position where you come to a critique of the initial conceptualizations. Many philosophers and metatheorists of social science have talked about a double hermeneutics. If I am investigating a subject matter, much of the subject matter consists in interactional dialogue between two subjects. These subjects will be hermeneutically negotiating with each other, encountering each other, and as they do so they will be trying to make sense of each other. This is the first hermeneutic. The second hermeneutic is me (the researcher) trying to make sense of their making sense of each other. This is only part of the subject matter of social science but it *is* part of it. It is important to recognize that if social science is in a hermeneutic relation with its subject matter then this is a two-way relation. Therefore, it is not just a question of the subject matter learning from us; we learn from it. Often, what we learn profoundly changes our own conceptual schemes and approach to life.

Some may not be entirely convinced that there is something more to social science than agents' conceptualizations. Take a speech action as an example: one person talking to another. What is it about this action that may escape my consciousness, in virtue of the corrigibility of my consciousness? First, we may not know much about the conditions for the speech act, such as how the two people came to be geographically in the same place, or why they are talking to each other.

We may be able to ask them what motivates them to speak, but aspects of their motivation may escape them, specifically their unconscious motivation. If we consider the tacit skills that they use in performing this speech act, as Noam Chomsky [1929–] has demonstrated, people are largely unaware of how it is that they do basic speech actions. Finally, there is the whole field of unintended consequences. Therefore, in general, any action is always conditioned by unacknowledged factors, unconscious motivation, tacit skills, and unintended consequences; and it is the role of social science to tell us about all that. Strictly speaking, there are no empirical regularities or constant conjunctions in social life. However, this does not mean that we cannot form law-like statements, such as that if you drink alcohol then you are more likely to drive badly. In this case, there is a causal mechanism that is well-acknowledged, namely that alcohol causes people to drive badly due to diminished cognition. However, even if you drive home after drinking and do not have an accident, the tendency that alcohol makes you a poor driver still exists. The alcohol will still have made you a worse driver; you would still have been safer driving home without it. Therefore, this mechanism may never manifest in a perfect sequence of events but this does not mean that the tendency does not exist. These are the kinds of law-like statements to which social science can aspire. They are tendencies and we cannot expect them to be reflected in a universal sequence of events.

This is basically the way that critical realism deals with the macro-dualisms of structure and agency, individualism and collectivism, and meaning and law. There is not enough space to go into all of the micro-dualisms, but we will briefly discuss how critical realism resolves the much-debated micro-dualism of facts and values. The dominant, mainstream position on facts and values is known as *Hume's Law*. It states that there is no way to get from a factual statement to a value statement. This is profoundly wrong and we can see that it is wrong when we consider that science is concerned with the criticism of (pre-existing) beliefs. Copernicus showed that the sun, and not the earth, is the centre of the solar system. This is an example of a characteristic of science, specifically, to criticize pre-existing beliefs. More generally, this characteristic is a feature of all factual discourse because there is not much point in repeating a factual statement to someone who already believes it. Therefore, all factual discourse is implicitly critical. However, when one criticizes a belief, one is also implicitly criticizing (evaluating, valuing) any action that is informed by that belief. For example, if someone claims that the sun does not go around the earth, they are also criticizing the actions informed by that belief. In the instance of Copernicus, the way that society at the time defined the calendar was incorrect due to the incorrect knowledge about the relationship between the earth and the sun. This resulted in the calendar becoming out of line with the seasons of the earth, something that greatly concerned Church leaders. To criticize the pre-existing belief was therefore also an evaluation or criticism of the actions derived from that belief and ultimately led to more appropriate actions given the objective at hand, namely to devise a calendar that did not get out of sync with the seasons.

Moreover, assuming as hermeneuticists do that central beliefs are characteristically part of their subject matter, then it is possible to show that a certain set of beliefs function in such a way as to uphold a particular institution. Returning to the Copernicus example, a consequence of Copernicus' theory was to demote the earth and therefore human beings from their position at the centre of the universe. This false belief – that the natural hierarchies of nature are a mirror of the natural hierarchies of human society – in part upheld the institution of the Church. We can therefore account for the Church's attachment to it because it supported the way that the Church justified its position at the top of the hierarchy of society. To criticize the false belief was to threaten the Church hierarchy, and hence Copernicus was accused of heresy and excommunicated. It is therefore apparent that if one determines that certain beliefs are false, then one is also bound into a critical relation with whatever it is that accounts for those beliefs. In a modern context, there are also certain beliefs that uphold certain social structures. For example, there is a belief that our value in society is linked to the kind of car that we drive; this supports the constant demand for expensive cars that supports the capitalist economy. To criticize this belief is also to criticize the capitalist economy. This opens up the possibility that social science has an emancipatory purchase on social life, including the life of the individual researchers involved (for a modern-day example of this, see Chapter 15).

Comparing the natural and social sciences

We now return to the critical realist discussion of the macro-dualisms. By resolving these dualisms we will have achieved certain of the conditions necessary to argue that social science is possible. However, we need to further consolidate our argument by looking systematically at the similarities and differences between the natural and the social. To begin with, we will look at the differences that social structures have from natural structures. The first difference is that we cannot perceive social structures directly. We can only perceive their effects; for example, we cannot actually perceive the capitalist economy. When we see a computer changing ownership, we do not perceive the capitalist economy; rather, we perceive one of its effects. However, this characteristic of social structures is not entirely unique to them because some natural structures like magnetic or gravitational fields are also not directly perceivable; we can only perceive their effects. If we can allow that some natural structures operate in this way, we can also allow that there are, or might be, social structures that operate in the same sort of way.

The second, radical difference between social and natural structures is that social structures only ever operate in open systems; they are always part of an open-system context. We cannot experimentally close these systems without violating them. This means that we cannot have predictive criteria for confirming theories/theorems in social science. We cannot have predictive criteria because we can only generate absolutely decisive test situations if we can close the system. If we cannot close the system, it is always possible that some other factor or event may occur to prevent a (true) prediction that otherwise would have occurred. For example, we might have a theory that racism is present in a large company and therefore predict that there will be few, if any, non-white directors. If, in fact, we find that there are several non-white Asian and African directors, this does not disprove our theory, as in an open system there may be confounding factors, such as that public pressure has resulted in the token appointment of non-whites. However, it is also possible that certain theories can seem to provide predictions in open systems, even when these predictions are simply artefacts of the open-system context. That is, it is illogical to infer causation from correlations in open systems. For example, it was found that infants who sleep with the light on are much more likely to develop myopia in later life. Statistically, it is therefore possible to say that we can predict the chances of a child developing myopia if we look at whether or not they sleep with the light on. It was therefore widely assumed that sleeping with the light on *causes* myopia. However, a later study at Ohio State University did not find that infants sleeping with the light on caused the development of myopia. It did find a strong link between parental myopia and the development of child myopia, also noting that myopic parents are more likely to leave a light on in their children's bedroom (Stone, Maguire and Quinn, 2000). In this case, the cause of both conditions – sleeping with the light on and myopia – is parental myopia, and the previously stated conclusion that sleeping with the light on causes myopia is false.

Although we cannot have predictive criteria to confirm theories/theorems in social science, it does not follow that therefore we cannot have explanatory criteria. We already use such explanatory criteria in social science. For example, after a certain event, we can sometimes see what it was that explains that event. Take the instance of the 2008 economic crash; afterwards, we could see that certain banks' lending behaviour explained what had happened. Furthermore, law-like statements in social science are more or less confirmed by other instances. For instance, there is the classic case of the law-like statements that relate to the formulation of suicidal tendencies in a person. These are more or less confirmed by a whole body of data. Similarly, we might have certain assumptions about the structure of national economies and capitalism which are more or less confirmed by a set of data.

In social science, we are always dealing with an open system and therefore confirmation and falsification depend on context. In reality there is never only "event and mechanism" or "agent and mechanism or structure"; there is also context. Therefore, in reality we have "agent, context, and mechanisms or structures". This is because the same mechanism or structure will act in a different way in a different context. It therefore follows that context becomes very important in our theories. The CA(I)MO model of explanation is useful here. It states that the features that we need for an explanation in general in social life include: context C, agent A, mechanism M, and outcome O. Therefore, CAMO is the basic model. However, if we are concerned with policy or intervention, then we need to add I: the social intervention. This is the CA(I)MO model of explanation.

Up to now, we have been looking at epistemological differences between social and natural structures, but what about the ontological differences? Ontologically there are four very important differences. These are:

1. Activity dependence – social structures are dependent on human activity in a way in which natural structures are not. Gravity does not depend on human beings, but capitalism does.
2. Concept dependence – social structures cannot operate independently of some conceptualization by agents, they are concept or belief dependent.
3. Space time dependence – social structures are more space time dependent in general than natural structures.
4. Internal relationality – as a social scientist, one's beliefs about the subject matter may themselves be a part of the subject matter. Or looking at it in another way, the social scientist and the philosopher of social science are part of, are immersed in, society. They are a part of their subject matter and this means that social scientists have to be reflexive in a way that natural scientists do not have to be.

What does this mean, in terms of whether or not we can do good social science? We *can* have confirmation and falsification of our social theories, provided that these are based on explanatory, rather than formally predictive, criteria. A great asset of social science is the hermeneutical moment which means that we already have agents' conceptualizations to give us a provisional account of a subject matter; in the natural sciences, our subject matter cannot speak to us. One way in which both natural and social scientists are similar is that they both argue in a transcendental way (retroductively). They therefore ask: What must be the case for a certain activity or event to be possible? Thus Marx asked the retroductive question: What must be the case for commodity production to be possible? What must be the case for there to be a society in which things are bought and sold? Durkheim (2005/1897) asked the retroductive question: What must be the case for suicides to be possible? This fundamental, retroductive mode of thinking is characteristic of all science. In so far as social science starts from conceptualized activities, it has a lot in common with philosophy. The hermeneutical component, combined with a retroductive investigation or procedure, allows a conceptual analysis of what is happening in a particular society. We can therefore ask: What must be the case (in terms of beliefs or conceptualizations) for a particular institution or aspect of society to be possible?

A toolkit for social scientists

In this chapter, we have described how critical realism argues for the conditions of the possibility of social science. In summary, critical realism concludes that social science *is* possible; and that it is possible in virtue of its differences from the natural sciences. Given that this is the case, how should we go about our work as social scientists? We suggest the following toolkit, illustrating it with a research project by Skinningsrud (2007) that looked at the development of the educational system in Norway.

1 Be a realist

You need to be a realist about your subject matter. That is, you need to think that *something* has happened, or that *something* is there; and that that *something* has an existentially intransitive reality. In terms of the educational system of Norway, the structures and mechanisms of the state and the religious establishment that enables them to exercise control over the schools are real. Skinningsrud's theory about them is not just a fictional "mental model".

2 Be a scientist

How are you going to investigate this real subject matter that exists independently of your investigation? You are going to want to investigate it scientifically. What does this mean from the point of view of critical realism? It means that you are going to be looking at generative mechanisms and structures, using retroduction (which is a characteristic of all science). You are not just going to be concerned to unearth patterns of events; you are going to try to explain these patterns by reference to a deeper reality of structures and mechanisms. This means that you are going to arrive at transfactual theories that explain the evidence. In this case, Skinningsrud used retroduction to arrive at a theory about the way that the reformation in Norway had important consequences for education, in which the role of the church was reduced and the role of the state increased. Her theory was not the only one, however, and she had to use judgemental rationality to decide amongst the competing theories; one theory, for instance, differed in terms of the role played by the Norwegian King in managing the schools before the reformation.

3 Be interdisciplinary

You are going to make use of the distinction between open and closed systems. This means that you are going to understand that your subject matter – in this example, the development of the Norwegian education system – will in all probability be constituted by a multiplicity of mechanisms drawn from perhaps radically different fields. Therefore, even though you might be a sociologist, you will need an interdisciplinary approach. In the case, Skinningsrud also had to play the roles of historian, political-economist, geographer, theologian, and constitutional lawyer, amongst others.

4 Employ hermeneutics

You are going to want to investigate your subject matter hermeneutically. Skinningsrud looked for historical documents that allowed her to read the writings of people historically involved in the educational transformations. If it had been possible, she would have spoken to people about their schooling. She read scientific works done on educational systems in other countries. She considered the scientists' theories and whether they applied to her data. Where these theories failed to explain what she was seeing, she had to either arrive at new theories or correct the old ones.

5 Make use of the TMSA

Since your subject matter is something which will exemplify social science, you are going to have to look at social structures and agencies. Therefore, it is likely that you will need to make use of the TMSA to allow you to theorize the way that agents reproduce and transform structures; while structure acts back on the agents and provides them with an enabling or constraining framework for their actions. In the TMSA, there are four planar aspects of social being and these will come into the analysis somewhere. Skinningsrud used a variation of the TMSA, the idea of morphogenesis, developed by the critical realist Margaret Archer (2010).

6 Think in terms of scale

You will also have to choose the appropriate levels of scale to operate on. Skinningsrud considered the educational system in particular localities of Norway, but also looked at features relating to the country as a whole, then the country in the context of other western European countries, and in principle, in terms of the global system of states. She gradually built up a picture of what accounted for the peculiarities of the development of the Norwegian educational system. At the broader scales, it was important for her to remember that a universal transfactual, such as the way that the reformation had certain implications for the educational systems throughout Europe (Archer, 2013), was not necessarily falsified because Norway was unique compared to other European countries and therefore did not always match their experience exactly. The changes to the educational systems in the European countries were still explainable in terms of the effects of the reformation, even though these effects were differentially experienced in each country due to other open-system factors.

The contemporary version of natural science is associated with practice that is more or less adequate, but nevertheless its philosophy (or theory) of science is inadequate. Therefore, the aim of critical realism is to provide a better or more adequate account of, or theory of, scientific practice. However, in the social sciences, much of the practice is itself flawed. This is at least partly because of (a) the problem of applying inadequate natural science theory to a social science context, which shows up its flaws; and (b) the aporetic consequences of the plethora of conflicting and inadequate alternatives to natural science theory. Therefore, in the social sciences, the aim of critical realism is the transformation of our practice in an appropriate way, guided by scientists' improved understanding and self-understanding. In other words, critical realist philosophy aims to enhance reflexivity and/or transform practice. In this chapter, we have tried to give you a toolkit to do this. In the next chapter, we will show how this toolkit can be radically deepened.

6

THE ONTOLOGICAL CASE FOR INTERDISCIPLINARITY

In the previous chapter, we presented the basic concepts of critical realism and discussed the characteristics of natural and social sciences, their similarities and differences. In this chapter, we will directly broach the main topic of this book, which is critical realism and interdisciplinarity. This is another way of saying that we will discuss applied critical realism, which in the social sciences always includes interdisciplinarity. To begin with, it is important to stress that one's methodology and abstract theorems – which we described in Chapter 5 – always have a double specificity. First, they must be specific to the research process and the progress that contemporary science has already made, or the contemporary status quo of the science. Second, they must be specific to the subject matter because one cannot apply abstract philosophy to any concrete reality without further arguments.

The argument that we are going to consider in this chapter concerns interdisciplinarity. When we (Roy Bhaskar and Berth Danermark) first started working on critical realism and interdisciplinarity, we were struck, as discussed in Chapter 2, by the fact that most of the literature reflecting the contemporary status quo of interdisciplinarity was not very deep in a philosophical sense and that it was almost entirely epistemological. In other words, there were no explanations as to what it is about the nature of the world that makes interdisciplinary work possible and indeed, as we are going to argue, necessary. As already explained, this failure to disambiguate the epistemological and ontological is highly problematic. It is important to ask whether or not one is concerned with an epistemological or an ontological issue or argument. In this chapter, we aim to remedy this situation by giving an outline of critical realism's main ontological arguments for interdisciplinarity.

Recall the nature of the world indicated by the new ontology that we described in Chapter 3, specifically the distinction between: (a) structures and events; and (b) open and closed systems. Consider how an experimental laboratory context is an artificial one. When scientists set up an experiment, they aim to isolate mechanisms from the influence of the open system. That is, they isolate individual mechanisms from other mechanisms and structures that potentially interact and compete with them. Therefore, in an experiment, a scientist studies the effect of a single mechanism working in isolation from the rest of nature. This is an artificial situation but it allows the scientist to generate a constant conjunction of events (empirical invariance) in a closed system. This kind of closed-system context occurs in nature in a few situations. For example, in an astronomical context, the solar system can be regarded as being effectively closed, but only if we look at the current time span, of perhaps a million years. If we want to go back 10 million years, then the system is not closed. Therefore, ultimately, everything in nature is part of an open system. From the point of view of the context with which most of us are concerned, strictly closed systems are only found in laboratories. Outside the laboratory, there are more or less open systems in which mechanisms are always working alongside each other. To put this more simply: in open systems you are always working with a multiplicity of causes; in a laboratory experiment, you have a single cause and you describe it very precisely.

The DREI(C) and the RRREI(C)

In Chapter 4, we briefly mentioned the DREI(C). This is the critical realist model of pure scientific activity or scientific activity which moves from one level of reality to another in concrete detail. However, critical realism suggests a different logic of scientific discovery for applied research: the RRREI(C) model. While the logic of retroduction features centrally in the DREI(C), the logics of abductive redescription and retrodiction are central to the RRREI(C) model (Bhaskar, 2008b/1993: 133). When scientists want to explain why events happen in the *open systemic world* – characterized as it is by a conjunctive multiplicity, rather than a disjunctive plurality of causes – they need the RRREI(C) model. In this model, the first R stands for the *resolution* of the complex event or phenomenon into its components, involving a conjunctive multiplicity of causes (i.e. a *and* b *and* c, etc.); the second R for the abductive *redescription* or recontextualization of these components in an explanatorily significant way; the third R for the *retrodiction* of these component causes to antecedently existing events or states of affairs; E for the *elimination* of alternative competing explanatory antecedents; I for the *identification* of the causally efficacious antecedent (or antecedent complex); and C for the iterative *correction* of earlier findings in the light of this (albeit provisionally) completed explanation or analysis.

Consider a simple event in an open system, like someone arriving late for a lecture one morning. In general, looking at the first R, there will be a multiplicity of causes – a multiplicity of factors – responsible for that event. In order to give a concrete explanation of that event, it is necessary to *Resolve* it into its components, i.e. we must look at all the causes or all the significant, relevant causes of the event. The second thing it is necessary to do for each cause is to find the best possible description – the most significant description of it. If we think about why someone was late, we might *Redescribe* the lateness as: "the trains weren't operating". This would be more relevant than redescribing the event in terms of the physical laws that were in operation. Therefore, one gives the best description, which is also the most relevant description. Then on the basis of that description it is necessary to *Retrodict* back to antecedent states of affairs or events that were responsible for the trains not working (the lateness), using one's knowledge of natural and social laws. In principle, there may be many reasons why the trains were not running on the morning that the person was late. Perhaps there was a strike, or perhaps there was a breakdown in the signalling system; but there may have been many other reasons too. Therefore, it is necessary, after each retrodictive moment, to *Eliminate* other alternative possible causes. Furthermore, supposing that it was a strike, we might ask what caused the industrial action. Therefore, there will be a multiplicity of causes and it will be necessary to repeat the RRRE until one has *Identified* a detailed picture of the causal genesis of the particular event that one wants to explain. Once this has been achieved, it may be necessary to *Correct* the overall picture in the light of the fuller and deeper knowledge. Eventually, this process will allow the inquirer to paint a detailed picture of what caused the lateness, or a bridge to collapse or a relationship to break up, or whatever it is that needs explaining.

However, the RRREI(C) presents something of a challenge for social scientists, in comparison to natural scientists. Natural scientists can usually apply already available, independently validated, generally accepted theory to explain their measurements. However, this is frequently not the case for social scientists, as there is often no theoretical knowledge available; and, even if theory is available, the open-system context in which social scientists must work means that they won't be able to apply the theory in a straightforward, uncomplicated, uncontested way. In part this is because, when we begin our research in the social world, even if we know *what* the mechanism is, we cannot know in advance *how* it will operate in the specific context concerned. This often leads to a simultaneous occurrence of the DREI(C) (retroductive theoretical discovery of mechanisms) and the RRREI(C) (retrodictive application of these theories), making it difficult to distinguish between the two, except analytically. It suggests the need for a *theorem of the contingent duality (and simultaneity) of discovery and application*, which, together with the *theorem of the (again contingent) co-incidence of retroductive and retrodictive moments in research* implies that the use of critical realism in the open-systemic world is potentially (or at least readily brings about) a creative process of discovery.

If we separate the retroductive and retrodictive moments in time, it is possible to build a unified general model that includes the following components:

> Resolution, abductive Redescription, Retroduction (RRR)
> Inference to the best explanation – most likely mechanism or complex (I)
> Retrodiction, Elimination, Identification of antecedents, and Correction (REI(C)).

This gives us the RRRIREI(C) model of exploratory investigation (see also Danermark et al., 2002: 109–111; Steinmetz, 1998: 170–186; Bhaskar, 2016: 81–82). These different types of discovery logic form the backdrop to our discussion of interdisciplinarity.

The stages of interdisciplinarity

The implication for social research of the nature of causal determination in an open system is that it must include the following interdisciplinary stages:

1. The first stage – a multiplicity of causes

    This ontological stage is implied by the open-system status of the world.

2. The second stage – a multiplicity of mechanisms or structures

    This ontological stage becomes necessary because, when we talk about causes in science, what we are concerned with are mechanisms or structures; and since we have a multiplicity of causes, we therefore have a multiplicity of mechanisms or structures.

3. The third stage – a multiplicity of theories

    This epistemological stage is necessary because the multiplicity of mechanisms or structures requires that we have a multiplicity of theories, each corresponding to the different mechanisms or structures. At this point, because this stage is essentially an epistemological one, a certain technical knowledge comes into play.

4. The fourth stage – a multiplicity of disciplines

    This epistemological stage is necessary because – while it is possible to imagine that one could explain a physical event using a multiplicity of theories about the physical causes, that is, it might be explicable in terms of one discipline, such as physics – nevertheless, in a social context, when there are a multiplicity of theories about a variety of mechanisms and structures, the theoretical explanation is likely to extend beyond the single discipline, and into multiple disciplines.

Therefore, one moves from: causes; to mechanisms; to theories; to disciplines. We might now ask: What necessitates a multidisciplinary approach to concrete phenomena in the world? Multidisciplinarity is needed because of emergence. Emergence occurs when one level of reality is radically emergent from another. For example, mind is emergent from body. When emergence is a factor, then we must use different disciplines, since we have to talk about social and psychological things as well as physical and chemical things. A well-recognised example of emergence is the mind from the body; similarly, society is emergent from individual people. When there is a strong argument for emergence then it is necessary to have different disciplines. In the case of mind emerging from body, this suggests the need for (at least) the disciplines of psychology and neurobiology; in the case of society emerging from individual people, this suggests the need for (at least) the disciplines of social science and psychology. This establishes the multidisciplinary nature of the explanations for concrete phenomena. Having got this far, the limitation of the mono-disciplinary approach becomes apparent because, if everything outside the laboratory has to be understood in terms of the multiplicity of causes, mechanisms, and theories, then arguably it has to be understood in terms of more than one discipline. This means that, when we are dealing with a reality that is complex, different disciplines are going to be involved. However, multidisciplinary is not the same as interdisciplinary. In a multidisciplinary approach, the different mechanisms are described in the language of the different disciplines and then they are summed up, listed, or enumerated. But what makes interdisciplinary work necessary is the fact that there are emergent outcomes. Scientists arrive at something qualitatively new. It is no longer possible to simply add up the results of the different disciplines. Scientists must do genuinely creative work between the disciplines. Interdisciplinarity is fundamentally implied by the prevalence of open systems and the emergence of levels and of outcomes.

However, there is also a dialectic here, in that there is a move from the necessity for interdisciplinary activity, to the necessity for intradisciplinary activity. Until this point we have assumed that the interdisciplinary mechanisms implicated in the explanation of the open-systemic phenomenon are themselves unaltered by their new emergent context. However, if we consider certain phenomena, such as the production of sounds or marks in human speech and writing, it is clear that this is often not the case; the mechanisms implicated may themselves be radically altered by the emergent synthesis or combination. When the mechanisms change, and are thus emergent, we can talk of intradisciplinarity. For this reason, not only are there different ontological laminations due to emergence between the disciplines, but there are also ontological laminations due to emergence within the disciplines (intradisciplinarity).

What we have done so far is to provide a sketch of the way that the (ontological) open-system nature of reality results in a multiplicity of causes which, if we are to have an understanding of it, necessitates multidisciplinarity, interdisciplinarity, and intradisciplinarity. We now turn to epistemological considerations and ask: How do we achieve new interdisciplinary theory that explicates how the qualitatively new outcome emerges? Or, how are we going to arrive at an understanding – in an interdisciplinary way – of the production of a new kind of working mechanism? This is where one has to introduce the concept of transdisciplinary work. When we talk about something new in science, what we are doing is talking about how it is that one can produce – epistemologically – a knowledge which has not been dreamt up or thought about before. Typically, one very useful way to begin to do this is to build models based on past cognitive successes in other disciplines and fields. So creative scientists are a bit like cognitive magpies, picking up interesting resources (in the form of analogies, metaphors, and models) wherever they can find them in order to construct an explanation that fits with the new kind of reality they have unearthed. This dovetails with the main epistemological argument for interdisciplinarity, which is its usefulness in scientific creation; it scaffolds the genesis of new ideas.

There is also the notion of crossdisciplinary research or inter-professional cooperation. Crossdisciplinarity, as we define it here, is the ability and the potential to empathize with, understand, and employ the concepts of disciplines and fields other than one's own. Such crossdisciplinarity is vital for successful interdisciplinary work at the epistemological level as members of the interdisciplinary team must be able to communicate effectively with each other in crossdisciplinary understanding. This, together with the need for creative transdisciplinarity, necessitates types of education and socialization of the interdisciplinary research worker that are significantly different from those currently found in orthodox monodisciplinarity.

To summarize our basic argument, we move from: open systems; to the necessary complexity of concrete reality; through to different levels of emergence; leading to multidisciplinarity; then interdisciplinarity and intradisciplinarity. Epistemologically, all of this implies a transdisciplinarity moment. The temporal logic of this process is outlined in Figure 12.1.

What does this mean in concrete detail? It means that reality is constituted by several different levels. To describe these levels, we use terminology first proposed by Andrew Collier (1989): the idea of a laminated system (for examples of laminated systems, see Table 6.1). Bhaskar and Danermark (2006) looked at the history of disability research and it seemed that the approaches were entirely, up to that date, actualist, monodisciplinary, and reductionist. It is likely that this was the case because these approaches were based on standard philosophy. Standard philosophy states that reality can be explained by reference to universal laws, but it defines these universal laws in terms of constant conjunctions: thus, whenever you have *a*, then you have *b*. However, this is not the case in open systems. For example, when

TABLE 6.1 Examples of critical realist interpretations of laminated systems

Bhaskar and Danermark's (2006) "interacting, coalescing" laminations or levels required to understand phenomena within the discipline of disability studies	1 Biological, more specifically, physiological, medical, or clinical mechanisms 2 Psychological mechanisms 3 Physical mechanisms 4 Psycho-social mechanisms 5 Cultural mechanisms 6 Socioeconomic mechanisms 7 Normative mechanisms
Brown's (2009: 23) "relational, laminar and emergent" critical realist model developed to understand phenomena within the discipline of education, and inspired by Bhaskar and Danermark's (2006) equivalent model for disability studies	1 Biological mechanisms, e.g. adequate nutrition 2 Physical mechanisms, e.g. classroom lighting 3 Psychological mechanisms, e.g. student motivation 4 Socio-cultural (including moral and political) mechanisms, e.g. parental beliefs about education 5 Normative mechanisms, e.g. as determined by curricula
Parker's (2010: 209) laminated system, illustrating the "emergence and dependency" of systems	Cosmological systems > life support systems > human material systems > human social systems > human cultural systems

you sit on a chair, despite the universal law of gravity, you do not fall to the ground. This is because, although you have a (the law of gravity) you do not have b (falling to the ground) and this is owing to the existence of other forces. Typically, in this case, you do not fall to the ground because a floor has been built where you are sitting. Therefore, reality cannot be modelled in an actualist way. However, when we looked at pre-existing disability research we found that in general the approaches had been reductionist or monocausal, based on this standard philosophical assumption that universal laws are constant conjunctions. For instance, in the early 1960s, the clinical or medical model dominated, in which disabilities were regarded as being rooted in the body, i.e. physical; hence, at this time, it was assumed that disabilities were the result of a physical set of causes. That is, the universal law was assumed to be: if a (certain physical attributes) then b (certain disabilities). As a reaction to this, in the later 1960s and in the 1970s, people regarded the source of disabilities as being socio-economic (the so-called Social Model). The idea here was that one only had a disability if there was an absence of the appropriate resources. If someone could not walk, it was only a problem if buildings were not fully wheelchair accessible. In the Social Model, disability was analysed in terms of accepted economic conditions and causes. That is, the universal law was assumed to be: if a (absence of economic conditions) then b (presence of disabilities). In the 1980s there was a reaction against the Social Model in terms of the "Foucauldian" model, named after Michel Foucault [1926–1984]. Here the idea was that disabilities were all a question of language, or how one talked about reality. That is, the universal law was assumed to be: if a (presence of certain language constructions) then b (presence of disabilities). The problem with these three approaches was not that they were false, because they all undoubtedly cast light on the nature and complex phenomena of disabilities, but rather that they were all partial. Instead, what was needed was some notion of reality that included medical, socio-economic, and cultural/linguistic practice. In other words, we needed to have a notion of a reality that is constituted by different levels. In Bhaskar and Danermark (2006), we argued for this in terms of disability research. Specifically, we argued for the idea of a laminated system which is constituted not purely by physical levels of reality, but also by biological or physiological, psychological, socio-material or socio-economic, cultural, and ethical levels of reality. We also included a socio-psychological level which was constituted by the dynamics of people involved, and a micro-sociological level. All of these levels are necessary to understand any concrete phenomena in disability research. An example of the laminated system-approach is that it can explain the difficulties that persons with disabilities have in trying to obtain, and keep, a job. In many industrialized countries, persons with reduced work capacity are excluded from the labour market. There is a reductionist tendency to explain this in medical terms alone. We call this approach the *medicalization* of a bio-psycho-social problem. Instead of such causal reductionism, we need to investigate holistic causality, since there are mechanisms at all levels influencing a person's position in the labour market.

This is the basic model needed to think about explanation in an open-systemic world. It requires contributions from interdisciplinary teams of researchers. In any particular research project there will be different laminated systems, and therefore how the researcher actually constructs the laminated system must reflect this specificity. We call this a conjunctive multiplicity; and we differentiate conjunctive multiplicities from disjunctive pluralities. A conjunctive multiplicity is simply the case that one is always going to have *this* and *that* and *something else* when explaining a phenomenon. However, a disjunctive plurality is what exists at the RRREI(C) stage of retrodiction, where there is a choice between one or more particular theories, which results in the necessity of the stage of elimination. Interdisciplinary research is not a question of a choice between one thing and another; it is a question of meshing different things into the explanatory schema. Does this mean that we cannot say anything more about a subject matter in an open system other than the fact that it is going to be constituted by a multiplicity of causes? No, this is just a starting point and to do so would be to commit eclecticism – where anything goes. To the contrary, the researcher hopes eventually to achieve a real definition of the subject matter. It may seem odd to talk here about a *definition*, when we have just been talking about *explanations*. This is because as science progresses, what is originally an explanation, if it is increasingly accepted as true, eventually becomes a definition. So, for example, the properties of water were originally explained as being due to the chemical characteristics of bonded hydrogen (H_2) and oxygen (O). However, we now define water as H_2O. In the case of a social situation, what today explains the existence of racism may tomorrow be the definition of racism. Bhaskar (2008b/1993: 110) writes: "After a further elapse of time the firmly established structure may be held to be definitional of a natural kind".

In our investigation into the case of disability research, we were able to arrive at a real definition of disability studies as an articulated lamination "in relation to the experience, and perception of the experience, of some impairment or functional loss, which itself or the effects of which, require to be socially or psychologically assessed, compensated (or accepted), transcended, mediated or otherwise reflected" (Bhaskar and Danermark 2006: 293). This was a tentative definition but it is what researchers ought to be able to do in their own fields of study. What one is trying to do in the context of interdisciplinary research is to avoid reductionism and monodisciplinarity on the one hand; and on the other hand to avoid eclecticism, simply calling everything, every cause, a level of reality (Brendel, 2003). However, one needs to have an idea of a contoured, shaped reality in which entities are interrelated and from there one can theorize a tentative, levels-of-reality, perspective.

Conditions for interdisciplinarity

Let us consider the necessary conditions for interdisciplinary research. First, interdisciplinary research requires the disambiguation of the ontological and epistemological to ensure clarity about the claims that one is making about the world.

Second, interdisciplinarity requires the closely related trio of metatheoretical unity, methodological specificity, and theoretical pluralism, which we can describe as follows:

- *Metatheoretical unity* is the philosophical, metatheoretical level, provided by critical realism, which provides notions such as: structures or mechanisms which are empirically verifiable or falsifiable; open and closed systems; and all the subsequent refinements and elaborations which we will discuss in later chapters.
- *Methodological specificity* is the idea that one's basic epistemology or methodology must be specific to a particular discipline. Therefore, although one has a metatheoretical perspective that is relevant to all the disciplines, nevertheless what one actually does is always governed by the nature of one's subject matter. For example, it is not possible to treat human beings, who have reasons for what they do, in exactly the same way that one can treat atoms.
- *Theoretical pluralism and tolerance* is the idea that researchers must be tolerant with respect to other disciplines. However, they may also have to be tolerant within their own discipline because a refuted theory or idea may become relevant in an interdisciplinary context. It may be that for many purposes a researcher might regard certain categories as inadequate but in a particular interdisciplinary context they may need to use them. Such tolerance is presupposed by methodological specificity since it is inevitable that researchers who are looking at different parts of the laminated system are going to have different ways of understanding and doing things.

Third, a condition for interdisciplinarity is that the educational process has to be modified. One likely difference in the educational process is that there will be more attention given to the case study. Take as an example a medical team, composed of doctors, psychologists, social workers, and nurses – all casting light on some particular aspect of reality. If they are working on, and thus describing, the same case, then there is a basis for commensurability between the different theoretical disciplines involved. Another likely difference in the educational process is that researchers will be educated in more than one base discipline; perhaps they will have two or three. For example, a researcher may not only have a major or MA in psychology but also in biology, physics, and environment science. This might reduce the feelings of alienation that many researchers report when working in an interdisciplinary context. Yet another possible difference in the education of researchers for interdisciplinarity is that, instead of educating researchers in subject-specific ways, they will be educated in methodologically specific ways. Thus, their researcher identity will be attached to their methodological skills, rather than the subject matter of their research. For example, consider two researchers – an educator and a psychologist – who are both using critical discourse analysis in their PhD research. Nevertheless, they see themselves as educator or psychologist first, and critical discourse analyst/practitioner second. However, it may be possible that in the future they will see themselves as critical discourse analysts first, and that the actual subject matter of their research will be secondary – resulting in their ability to move fluidly between disciplines, always bringing their particular methodological skills with them.

A fourth condition for interdisciplinary research is that we need to dissolve the professional barriers to it. Currently, interdisciplinary researchers are not valued in the same way as their monodisciplinary counterparts; for example, they risk losing out on funding and promotions (Clarke et al., 2011). We need to overcome these issues so that the interdisciplinary research worker is seen as making an important contribution to their home discipline. One way to do this is to truly celebrate the transdisciplinary moment of science. The most creative scientists in any field are likely to be those with experience in other fields as well.

From the point of view of critical realism, applied research must be interdisciplinary because phenomena occur in the open-system context of the world. This means that researchers are always dealing with a multiplicity of causes and hence with a multiplicity of mechanisms, theories, and potentially disciplines. As long as we have emergence then necessarily there will be different disciplines. When one is dealing with the human sciences, or any reality which is affected by human beings, then one is dealing with a reality that is emergent. One will therefore need at least two perspectives, or two disciplinary matrixes, to explain it. This is the critical realist explanation of interdisciplinarity and on the basis of this explanation we can say certain things about the way that interdisciplinary work should be carried out. We can say that the interdisciplinary research team should construct a laminated system consisting in a conjunctive multiplicity of levels or laminations of reality. This system should not be reductionist, neither should it be totally eclectic: it should provide a version of reality that is contoured and differentiating. Interdisciplinary research should also display the characteristics of the trio of metatheoretical unity, methodological specificity, and theoretical pluralism and tolerance.

7
THE SEVEN STEPS TO DEEPER UNDERSTANDING OF ONTOLOGY

The main barrier to metatheoretical unity, the cornerstone of successful interdisciplinarity, is an inadequate understanding of ontology. This chapter resolves this problem by re-vindicating the study of ontology for contemporary times. Earlier chapters provided a general conceptual overview of the different ways to develop the basic argument or basic concepts of critical realism, turning on: the argument for ontology and the argument for a new ontology; the distinctions between the transitive and intransitive dimensions; ontology and epistemology; and structures and generative mechanisms vs. patterns of events. This was followed by a discussion of the application of this general conceptual system to the field of the social sciences. However, there are other ways to develop or apply critical realism (this book is an example of such an application or development, since it focuses on concrete phenomena in the world such as health, wellbeing, and disabilities). In this chapter, we consider how critical realism can be developed in terms of deepening our understanding of ontology. Specifically, this process has seven steps:

1. The first step in the development of ontology thematizes being as such. It argues: (a) for the need for an ontology (being); and (b) that this being is structured and non-identical, in other words, being has a structure and contains differences. These are essential categories for understanding phenomena in the world, but they lead to others. The publication of Bhaskar's (2008b/1993) book *Dialectic: The Pulse of Freedom* ushered in a new phase of critical realism, called dialectical critical realism. Here, Bhaskar added the next three steps in the re-vindication of ontology (steps 2–4 below).
2. The second step thematizes being as processual, as changing, and understands change as presupposing absence. Here, we have concepts of negativity, negation, contradiction, absence, process, rhythm, rhythmic, space, and time.

3. The third step understands being as a totality, or a whole, and involves the analysis of categories such as internal relations, holistic causality, and the concrete universal.

In steps 1–3, Bhaskar re-looked at the major categories of philosophical literature in the past and thematized them in a critical realist way, as ontological.

4. The fourth step looks at being as incorporating specifically transformative praxis, that is human action.
5. The fifth level of the critical realist ontology understands being as reflexive.
6. The sixth step understands being as meaningful, against the view of being as meaningless or nihilistic.
7. The seventh step emphasizes the priority of identity over difference and unity over antagonism and split.

Step 1: being (ontology) is unavoidable and layered

The first step of this development of critical realist ontology is the claim that there is no way to avoid ontology. Every system of thought designed to apply to the world presupposes something about the nature of the world. For instance, when Hume argued that causal laws are constant conjunctions of events, he presupposed that the world is flat, undifferentiated, and unchanging. Let us imagine having a conversation with a stereotypical postmodernist, who denies ontology:

POSTMODERNIST: You know; it is not true that you have to presuppose ontology. There is nothing in the world except language. Derrida (1998: 158) said that there is nothing beyond the text.[1] And therefore you do not have to do ontology; you do not have to have an assumption that the world has a certain form.

BHASKAR: Let us try to understand what you are saying. Are you telling me that all that there is, is language?

POSTMODERNIST: Yes, that is what I am telling you.

BHASKAR: From what you have said, you are at least claiming a certain ontology, since language, by your own admission, exists and therefore has an ontology. That is, you have admitted that the world has an ontology; namely, that it is composed of language. If you think that the world is linguistic, then you are making a substantive claim about the world.

POSTMODERNIST: No, this is not a substantive claim about the world, it is not saying anything. For example, Rorty (1982: 126–127) says that language is a tool rather than a medium – a concept is just the regular use of a mark or noise – language is just human beings using marks and noises to get what they want.

BHASKAR: Since you are not making a substantive claim, there is no reason why I should accept your speech action and respond to it because it is just a sequence of sounds. Unless you are actually making a claim about the world, unless you are prepared to admit that what you are saying is real, then no one needs to take your claim seriously. Therefore, if you want to be taken seriously, it is impossible to avoid an ontology of some form or another.

POSTMODERNIST: Quite right, there is no need to take what I say seriously, as Rorty (1989: 39) also said, we postmodernists emphasize the spirit of playfulness and (73) we are never quite able to take ourselves seriously.

We can therefore agree that if we want to be taken seriously, we must admit that ontology is unavoidable. However, as well as being unavoidable, ontology is also "all-inclusive". Ontology therefore includes epistemology. Since beliefs are part of being, then the very distinction between ontology and epistemology has to be seen as a distinction within ontology; after all, science is part of being. This also means that false scientific theories and false beliefs generally are part of being; it means that illusions are part of being. Think for a moment about the claim that vampires do not exist. What are we saying? We are saying that there is nothing in the world that roughly corresponds to vampires. However, the belief that there are vampires *is* nevertheless something that exists; we can safely say there are no vampires in the world but there *are* false beliefs that vampires exist. Therefore, illusions and false beliefs are part of the world; thus, we can say that they are ontological. As such, they have the power to affect us. For instance, if someone believes in vampires, they might have certain rituals to protect themselves from vampires, or try to avoid places where they think that vampires reside.

Dispositional realism

Another implication of a basic critical realism is dispositional realism. We easily understand that the actual is real; therefore, actual events, such as the attack on the World Trade Center in New York, are real. However, are possible events real? In critical realism, we say that they are and therefore, for instance, we can distinguish between real possibilities and illusory ones. Everything that is actual is an instance of the possible and therefore critical realists argue that the possible is a more basic category than the actual. Furthermore, the notion of real possibilities is essential to science and social life. This is because, when we assume that something is wrong in the world, we also assume that something else is possible in the world. That "something else" is a real possibility and this links to the strand of ethical thinking that critical realists call *concrete utopianism*. Concrete utopianism differentiates those possibilities that are real from those that are not. "Real" here means "realizable" and it applies to those possibilities that may be reliably actualized given particular constraints. Such constraints come in many forms. They may be physical, chemical, or biological; but they might also be social or economic. For instance, ecological (physical, chemical, and biological) constraints most likely preclude the achievement of the illusory utopia desired by many within the current consumerist approach to society; there are simply not enough natural resources for all human beings to achieve the level of wealth of the world's elite. Economic constraints might limit a family's choices in terms of the kind of housing that it may occupy, depending on the financial resources available to it. Social constraints might limit the kinds of relationships that certain people can have at a particular time, for instance in some societies it is currently legally impossible for people of the same sex to get married – although the possibility that this might change in the future is also a real one – and we might go so far as to say that globally there is a real tendency for same-sex marriage to be legalized. Therefore, this first step of the ontological development of critical realism implies dispositional realism; something is real if it is a possibility or a tendency. However, it also implies categorial realism.

Categorial realism

This is the idea that the categories of philosophy, or indeed categories in general, are themselves real. Most philosophers, following Immanuel Kant [1724–1804], think of categories of things such as law, causality, space, and time as things that we impose on the world. They think that there is an empirical "manifest" that we receive in sense perception and that we then impose these categories on the world. This is also Karl Popper's (2012/1945) methodological nominalist position. This position is unjustifiable because, for example, it assumes that we can have causes but not causation. However, if individual causes or causal laws exist, such as Ohm's law or Galileo's law, then the category "causation" also exists. Popper (2012/1945: 2030) explained his methodological nominalism in terms of puppies. He said that we can only ever describe individual puppies, and that it is not the business of science to ask the question, "What is a puppy?" For Popper therefore, there is no real category of "puppy", it is just something that we impose on the world. However, for critical realists there is a real category of puppy, although empirically every puppy that we meet will be an entirely unique individual example of the category "puppy". To disagree that categories are real results in the contradiction that philosophy is something that is apart from the world. Furthermore, for critical realists who disagree with categorial realism, the categories of philosophy (such as law, causation, time, and space) are not real. As with the conclusion of our discussion with the postmodernist, we conclude here that we cannot take the ideas about philosophy seriously since they are not about something real; they do not refer to the world itself. To the contrary, critical realism elucidates a philosophy that both is part of the world and refers to the world, including the most abstract features of that world.

The concept of truth

This first step in the development of critical realist ontology also includes the idea of realism about truth. Any full analysis of truth understands it as a multi-componential concept; there is no single concept of truth. Bhaskar (2008b/1993: 217) argues that truth has at least four distinct meanings, each of which presupposes the one before, and which we expand upon next: truth as fiduciary; truth as warrantedly assertable; truth as expressive referential; and truth as alethic.

1. Truth as fiduciary

   In everyday parlance, if someone makes the claim that something is true, what they normally mean is that we can trust what they say; we can rely on what they are saying. This is truth as fiduciariness.

2. Truth as warrantedly assertable

   This is the sense of truth that philosophers and epistemologists have customarily considered. One might argue that Einstein's theory is, in relation to Newton's theory, warrantedly assertable. Truth as "warrantedly assertable" is a judgementally rational aspect of a concept of truth that applies to the transitive dimension or epistemology.

3. Truth as expressive referential

   A third sense of truth leads us to say that the statement "the grass is green" is true. Here, what the speaker means is that the statement "the grass is green" is the most perfect expression that they can think of for the fact that the grass is green. This theory of truth is associated with the work of Alfred Tarski [1901–1983]. This is what we try to do in our speech action when we express the world. It is what we attempt to do with most of our statements.

4. Truth as alethic

   This sense of truth is fundamentally ontological and assumes ontological stratification. In this version of truth, there is a move from one ontological structural level to a deeper and more basic one, thereby giving the reason for, or ground of, something. The more basic structure is assumed to be the truth of the less basic structure. Therefore, we might argue that the alethic truth of green grass is that grass contains chlorophyll, which reflects the green component of the light spectrum. This more basic structure is part of ontology; it is what makes ontology stratified. Once we have this alethic concept of truth, then truth can, in a wider ontological sense, designate anything that makes a proposition true. In this way, the critical realist theory of truth includes a referential counterpart of the expressive use of truth.

It is important to consider the different kinds of truth because, as we mentioned in the first chapter, critical realism is committed to enhanced reflexivity which allows us to identify theory–practice inconsistencies. In many places in social life there are obvious theory–practice inconsistencies or contradictions. For instance, a scientist may in their experimental activity (their practice) presuppose that the world is structured and differentiated, but contradictorily their beliefs (their theory) may reflect an empiricist notion of the world as flat and undifferentiated. Therefore, the scientist has a false theory coexisting with a practice. However, any experimental scientist could not possibly carry out their work unless they acted on (remained faithful to the axiological necessity of) the alethic truth of the critical realist analysis of law, which requires a structured and differentiated world. Whenever they set up a laboratory experiment, effectively setting up an artificially closed system, they are presupposing that there are real transfactual laws that operate at a different level to actual reality. In other words, they are doing something epistemically necessary in setting up a laboratory situation; and such experimental procedures give them access to laws that can be applied transfactually. This is implicit in their practice, despite their denial of the existence of transfactual laws. The scientist unselfconsciously, for the most part, carries out the activities required to arrive at transfactual theories. At the same time, the theoretical or philosophical apparatus that denies the need for such practices runs idle, playing no role in the scientist's daily practice. It is ironic that the false belief in theory is sustained by the scientist's more adequate practice, and in virtue of this the theory–practice ensemble manages to sustain itself. In other words, reality contains axiological necessities, or imperatives, that must be satisfied, for any belief (or social situation) to continue. Of course, the aim of this critique is not to undermine the scientists but to say to them, "Look at this wonderful thing that you are actually doing!" In the process, the empirical scientist who happens to be an empiricist will understand that empiricism must give way to a more adequate philosophy of science along the lines of the critical realist analysis of laws based on an understanding of ontology as structured and differentiated.

TINA compromises and emancipatory discourse

Bhaskar (2008b/1993) called these contradictory theory–practice ensembles *TINA compromises* after Margaret Thatcher, whose nickname was TINA. This was due to her constant reiteration that *there is no alternative* to an economy based on monetarism, and yet the economy only continues because people satisfy certain axiological necessities of economic life that contradict monetarism. A TINA compromise is therefore the combination of false theory and adequate practice. It paves the way for what could be loosely called the logic of emancipatory discourse. Typically, in an emancipatory discourse, there is a level of reality which is basic and then there is another level of reality which shackles or suppresses that more basic level of reality. We can apply this to any emancipatory discourse, any discourse at all about freedom. Perhaps the most elaborately formulated emancipatory discourse is the discourse of Marxism. Here the basic level of reality is that human beings are essentially creative workers. However, this basic level of creativity is shackled by the class system and therefore the Marxist injunction is to overthrow the class system. In terms of the TINA compromise, the creativity of the worker is denied, and yet the system depends upon their creativity; there is an axiological necessity for it. According to this schema, the process of emancipation is therefore a process of shedding in order to stop shackling the more basic level. Emancipation is therefore simply (!) the removal of the constraints that prevent the more basic axiological necessity from being fully expressed. Therefore, emancipation is possible in the sense that there is already something present that is being shackled by something else (which needs to be shed).

The idea of emergence

These ideas – of dispositional realism, categorial realism, the different kinds of truth, TINA compromises, and emancipatory discourses – are some of the far-reaching implications of the simple idea at the first step in the critical realism development of ontology, namely that being is unavoidable and that it is structured and differentiated. Between the first step (being as structured) and the second step (being as process), we have the idea of emergence which we have already discussed in earlier chapters. In terms of emergence, one level of being will be qualitatively different from a more basic level. While the higher level is unilaterally dependent on the more basic one, it is nevertheless taxonomically irreducible to it. The higher level of being is also causally irreducible to the more basic level in the sense that it has the capacity to act back on the more basic level. However, there are two forms of emergence, both of which are important: the first form is superimposition emergence; and the second form is intra-position emergence. Superimposition emergence is the idea that the emergent level is the superstructure; intra-position emergence is the idea that the emergent level is formed within the more basic level. Whether the outcome is at the macro-level (a new type of structure) or at the micro-level (merely a structuratum), it normally remains heteronomously conditioned and controlled by the lower-order one – onto or into which it has been super- or intra-posed.

An example of superimposition emergence is the instance where human beings are both emergent from, and have discovered, physical laws, specifically mechanical and electrical laws, and use their knowledge to make cars. Thus, the car works by virtue of the mechanical and electrical laws that they have discovered. One could then argue that the human beings, through their product, the car, are determining the boundary conditions for the operation of certain mechanical and electrical laws. This is the superstructural level (a higher-order level) which is emergent from a lower-order level but which then acts on the lower-order level to provide it with boundary conditions.

An example of intra-position emergence is to be found in discussions of climate change. An illustration is Parker's (2010: 209) conception of ecological emergence, reproduced in Table 6.1. Intra-position emergence is present in the way that the ecological (life-support) level is formed within the cosmological level and then the human material level is formed (nested, embedded) within the ecological level and then the social level is nested within the human material level, and the cultural level similarly nested within the social level.

Step 2: being as process

The fallacy that is unearthed in the second step of the deepening (re-vindication) of ontology is the fallacy of supposing that there is nothing negative in the world. This fallacy (or doctrine) is called ontological monovalence by Bhaskar (2008b/1993). It is the idea that being has one value only, namely that of presence or positivity. This doctrine goes back to the pre-Socratic Greek philosopher Parmenides of Elea [515–460 BC] who said that you cannot say "not" – that there is no such thing as "not" – by which he meant that there is no such thing as "not" or "no" in reality. Plato [428–348 BC] was also convinced of this and he therefore analysed apparently negative qualities, such as change, in terms of purely positive qualities, such as difference. Let's think about what it means to say that there is no absence in the world. Imagine what a purely positive world would be like. It would be a world in which there was no space between us, nothing around us; there would be no emptiness. It would be a world in which there was no pause between the words that we utter and no space between the marks that we write. This world would be ridiculous! We need boundaries and we need space to make sense of anything. Material things could not exist unless they had spaces around them and spaces inside them. This is the most primitive form of absence, where there is nothing present. Furthermore, absence is ontologically prior to presence. A wider explanation of this claim is given in Bhaskar (2008b/1993). In terms of interdisciplinarity, it is enough to know that we need concepts of absence as well as concepts of presence and that being presupposes absence.

The reason that this is important is that if we want to change things (which one assumes we do) then we need to understand the process of change itself and in order to understand change it is necessary to realize that it presupposes absence. That is, it presupposes the coming into being of something and the passing away or the going out of being of something else. If a person is thirsty and takes a drink, then that thirst passes away. The absence that the person had – the sense of thirst – is satiated by the coming into being of a new state. This idea is the basic critical realist idea of change. Something new happens; there is a change. A previous state is transformed and a new state comes into being. There are some philosophers who dispute this version of change, such as the Platonists, the atomists, and the philosophical tradition. They would say that when something changes, this is because certain unchanging features or aspects of reality are recombined. They might say, in terms of atoms, that we only have unchanging atoms and that we only have the appearance of change because the atoms recombine in a different form. However, we know that before the *big bang* there were no atoms; therefore, new atoms do in fact come into being.

Dialectic

This second step in the deepening and re-vindication of ontology is allied with dialectic. Dialectic is associated with the philosophy of Georg Hegel [1770–1831]. Karl Marx [1818–1883] thought that Hegel was a great philosopher, who provided an outline of the basic form of dialectic, but who unfortunately shrouded it in mysticism. While it is true that Hegel made this mistake, his dialectic is nevertheless a stroke of genius in that it reveals a basic pattern of social progress, including progress in science. At any given stage of such progress, there is an absence or an incompleteness of some sort, and as the progress continues that absence is rectified. Thus, one moves from an incomplete situation to a more comprehensive totality. Hegel (1998/1807) described a threefold dialectic which starts from a position of identity, then moves through negativity to totality. Bhaskar (2008b/1993), however, formulated a critical realist dialectic which differs from Hegel's. In the critical realist version, one begins with: (1) a position of non-identity; then moves through (2) negativity; to (3) a different form of totality from Hegel's, one in which totality is open rather than closed; and then to (4) transformed praxis. The first, second, third, and fourth components of this dialectic are the first, second, third, and fourth steps of the seven steps of the deepening – re-vindication – of ontology elaborated within this chapter. Bhaskar (2008b/1993) named these four steps as follows: 1M first moment; the second step 2E second edge; the third step 3L third level; and the fourth step 4D fourth dimension (MELD). Nevertheless, despite the differences, Hegel's fundamental vision remains in the critical realist version. What excited Marx was the way that Hegel had identified an indispensable mechanism of the advancement of science, whereby:

> Incompleteness → inconsistency → movement to greater totality (that is, a more inclusive or comprehensive theoretical or social situation).

Dialectic in science

According to Kuhn (2012/1962), normal science does not proceed as we might expect. It is not a question of a scientific neophyte testing the theory to see if it is true or false; rather the scientific community tests the neophyte to see that they have got what it takes to make the theory true, to confirm it (perhaps in a new context). However, after a period of time the anomalies that always exist in normal science abound; they grow greater and greater and after a period of time they are so great that science moves into a new phase which is a phase of revolution. Revolutionary science continues until there is a new concept or a new theory, a new world view, which avoids the anomalies. The scientific community then embarks on a period of relative consistency again. From a critical realist perspective, what happens at the first stage is that the anomalies reach a point where you need to discover something new about reality – a deeper structure, aspect, or width of reality – a deeper degree of totality. This conceptual breakthrough allows the scientist to restore consistency. Therefore, at the basic level, there is a theory which is more or less adequate but, like all theories, it has left something out. That which is left out results in an absence or incompleteness of the theory which eventually reveals itself in the form of anomalies or inconsistencies. The accumulation of inconsistencies continues until some bright theorist sees what is left out. The deeper level of structure, that was of course there all along, is thus discovered and put back into the theory. In this way, scientists restore consistency to their work. This is a dialectical process in which the incompleteness of theories is gradually and progressively rectified by greater and greater completeness, leading to more comprehensive totalities. For example, Einstein came along and discovered relative space time. He added this into the existing Newtonian mix, resulting in a more comprehensive view of totality where there are a different form of space time and a different form of mass and energy. In another example, we might argue that our current, mainstream theory of economics is experiencing anomalies and inconsistencies due to the absence of the environment from the theory.

Dialectic in society

This idea of dialectic – the move from incompleteness or absence to greater completeness or totality – can help us to make sense of progress in society. An example might be the process by which women in the UK were given the vote (suffrage). Originally, there was an absence, because the body politic was constituted only by men. Obviously, something important was left out, the women, but by giving them the vote this absence was removed, restoring the situation to greater completeness. Similarly, certain countries such as Britain, France, Germany, Italy, Belgium, Portugal, and Spain had empires; and what was left out of the suffrage was the rights of the people who were the subjects of these empires. This was followed by decolonization after the Second World War, when there was a massive increase in the world politic as countries like India and countries in Africa became part of it. It can therefore be argued that some changes in social life approximate to a dialectical model in which progress occurs by rectifying incompleteness in an original position.

However, it is important to note that not all change is like this. Besides dialectical change, there is also entropic change. In entropic change, the absence or the incompleteness is not rectified but is increased; thus, coherence decreases in entropic change. The second law of entropy says that the universe goes towards increasing disorder; it is thus anti-dialectical. In any particular situation, it is an empirical question as to which way the changes are going to go.

Dialectic as the axiology of freedom

One might ask: Why is it important to think of the dialectic in terms of absence and absenting? This is because every intentional act, everything that one might want to do, can be put into a negative or absented form. If someone is trying to achieve something, perhaps they intend to do something or they want something, then they are trying to rectify an absence in the world. Let us say that they are hungry and therefore they go for lunch. In this instance their intentional activity is directed at remedying or rectifying an absence or incompleteness, namely the lack of food in their body. Through their intentional actions, they are trying to absent an absence, get rid of an absence, by filling it with a presence. This application of the dialectic resulted in the recursive definition of freedom as absenting absence and it is why Bhaskar (2008b/1993) called dialectic "the axiology of freedom".

Dialectic and contradiction

Contradiction is a very important category in the critical realist toolkit as it helps us to identify absence, and identifying absence is essential to the process of taking steps towards change. However, some philosophers say that there are no contradictions in the world (e.g. Priest, Beall and Armour-Garb, 2004). If they had said that there are no *logical* contradictions in the world then we would agree with them. There are no logical contradictions outside thought because it is only within thought that logic holds. However, there certainly are contradictions in the world. For example, a sustainable world is inconsistent with, or in contradiction to, our current levels of fossil fuel use. Contradictions can and should motivate agents towards their resolution because if they are left unresolved the situation is likely to degenerate further. In the case of climate change, we need to resolve the contradiction of our use of fossil fuels or we are likely to face severe consequences.

Dialectic as process

Dialectic helps us to better understand process. To be able to fully appreciate process, we need to think more deeply about space and time, as many social scientists are now beginning to do. For instance, to better understand a city it is helpful to see it as being the presence of the past. If we look at the buildings all around us, we see that they come to us from the past. Think of the traditions that you inhabit; they too are the presence of the past. Our social life is saturated with the presence of the past. Many features of social life have this processual nature; we can see them as a sort of rhythmic, or flow. Indeed, we can understand our own life in terms of these rhythms or flows. Because products are easier to see, we tend to forget about the processes. However, we need processes-in-products because we need to be able to look at the totality constituted by the interplay of processes. We also need products-in-process, such as individual human beings, who are products of their past but they are also in the process of making their future.

These ideas – dialectic in science and society, dialectic as the axiology of freedom, the role of contradiction in dialectic, and dialectic as process – are the second level of ontology, where we consider being as process. The key or root concept here is absence. We now move to the third step in the critical realist development of ontology.

Step 3: being as totality

This is the level of internal relations. Things can be related to each other both internally and externally. A is internally related to B if, and only if, it would not act in the way that it characteristically does unless B was related to it. We say that this relationship is symmetrically internal if this condition also applies reciprocally, and therefore B also needs to be related to A for it to act the way that it characteristically does. The internal relationality of something depends on whether some other, related, thing affects its identity. In cases of thoroughgoing internal relationality, we intuitively think of the structures "interpenetrating" each other and as forming a "totality". However, causal structures may interact in a normic or a systematic way without being internally related. Systems can therefore be divided into two types: "mechanical" complexes of externally interacting structures (such as billiard balls knocking into each other on a billiard table); and "organic" totalities of internally related intra-acting ones (such as the individuals in a family). Nevertheless, particular systems may have both types of connections; that is, pairs of structures (and their relations) may be related in both mechanical (external) and organic (internal) ways. It therefore follows that, even where structures coalesce or cohere as a totality, not all the causal interactions between them are internal (affect their identity). Existential parity (separation, such as two separate billiard balls) is compatible with ontological differentiation and depth because pervasive internality in a system is compatible with the differentiated and highly specific causal roles within it.

In the natural world, it is relatively simple and usual to treat objects separately or atomistically as distinct and self-contained individuals which interact mechanically. However, in the social world, the idea that it is always possible to treat objects atomistically collapses. For instance, the words in this sentence are internally related to the words in the last sentence. Societal roles are internally related to other roles (rely on them for their identity or their characteristic ways of behaving), such as the way that employers are internally related to their workers, teachers to students, and parents to children (in these examples, the pairs are symmetrically internally related). Bhaskar (2008b/1993) uses the term "holistic causality" to capture the way that internal relations may be developed and systematically understood. Holistic causality involves the way that internally related elements cohere as a whole. In terms of holistic causality:

a) The form of the combination causally co-determines the elements; and
b) The elements causally co-determine (mutually mediate or condition each other) and so causally co-determine the form of the combination.

At this level, therefore, one needs to think about things in a complex/contextual way. Ecologists since the 1960s and 1970s have been trying to think in terms of holistic causality, but in the absence of the idea that ontological reality is structured and differentiated, their claims have been deemed epistemologically weak. This is because mainstream empiricist scientists assume that deep ontological structures do not exist; they therefore assume that normic statements about such structures are merely "idealizations" or "abstractions". For such empiricist scientists, only events or experiences are truly real. As a result, ecologists like Scriven (1974: 222) are required to think of their normic statements as "guarded" generalizations. However, the conception or theory of the generative mechanism or structure that backs a normic statement need not be "idealized" or "abstract" since it refers to ontologically existing structures. If we assume that "theoretical" is a synonym for "unreal" (or at least "less real"), then normic statements appear as "ideal" in that the tendency or mechanism that they describe may be rarely if ever manifest in unmodified form due to the mediations associated with holistic causality. We touched on this in Chapter 4, when we explained how the fact that we are not falling to the ground does not suggest that we deny the existence of gravity. This is because mediations, such as the presence of the chair upon which we are sitting, prevent gravity from having this effect on our bodies. Just as we are unable to take seriously the post-modernists' claims about truth or the philosophers' claims about categories, if they are not about something real, so we cannot take seriously the empiricist ecologists' claims – their normic statements about the ecological systems of the planet – if they are not about something real. It is this contradiction that is exploited by climate change deniers who suggest that ecological theories about climate change are not scientific. For example, Philip Bratby (2010), in a speech to the House of Commons, stated that climate change science is questionable because, according to Karl Popper, "a theory should be considered scientific if and only if it is falsifiable" and that, "climate science is one in which in-situ experiments cannot be performed… In other words, the scientific methodology has been inverted…; a hypothesis was framed, and then data sought to confirm it rather than to falsify it". Therefore, for Bratby, climate science should not be taken seriously since normic statements about deeper structures and mechanisms have no reality, by which he means they are not falsifiable and cannot be experimentally tested.

However, when one makes a normic statement – such as that contemporary climate change is the result of human industrial activity – one is not making a guarded or idealized statement about an empirical reality. Rather one is making a statement about a different level of reality. This statement may be guarded or idealized in its own right, but not because it is, at best, a kind of empirical generalization. Normic statements are not empirical statements at all; they are about the ontological non-empirical level of reality, and they assume that reality is ontologically structured. In a similar way, social scientists make normic statements about, for example, the way that the economy works. However, without an acknowledgement of the ontologically real level of structures and mechanisms, social scientists, like the ecologists, remain vulnerable to the charge that their models are "just" models, or even that they are non-scientific (the implication being that one need not take them seriously). An example of this is provided by Tesh (1988: 169) who stated: "research that takes the social structure as the unit of analysis gets pushed to the periphery of science. At most it is a lesser kind of science – social science. At worst it is not science at all but a pseudoscience contaminated with politics". As a counter to such accusations, critical realism strengthens the claims of ecological and social scientists by insisting that their theories are about ontologically real things and therefore that they can be taken seriously. In contemporary policy contexts, if a politician does not like the implications of the content of a theory, such as the implications of the theory that climate change is anthropogenic, then they can simply say that it is "just a model" and that it is not based on proper science. To the contrary, a general understanding of the theory as being about something real insists that naysayers cannot dismiss it on such epistemological grounds. They would be forced to engage with the theory's content, that is, the adequacy of the theory to explain the empirical evidence. In the case of climate change, the theory that (at the moment) best explains the evidence is that human activity is the underlying reason for it.

The concrete universal

There is one other important concept at the third level, which is the idea of the concrete universal. Every universal that we come across in the world is a concrete universal. For example, every human being will incorporate both universal aspects of being a human and aspects that are not universal. Take the example of a specific kind of human, such as a woman. Every woman will contain four aspects, which are:

1. Every woman is a universal woman

    In virtue of being a woman, she will have certain characteristics in common with all other women.

2. Every woman is a mediated woman

    Nevertheless, in virtue of being a woman, she will also have certain characteristics in common with some but not all other women. These are her mediations, or her specificities.

3. Every woman has a geo-historical trajectory

    All women come from different places and different times; we all have a different trajectory. Perhaps the woman in question comes from Norway, China, Nepal, or the USA. However, her trajectory is not just geographical, it is historical, because women are born at different times.

4. Every woman is a unique individual

    But supposing that two women came from exactly the same place and were born at the same time, so they had exactly the same geo-historical trajectory; would they therefore be the same? No, and this is because there is a fourth level of analysis, namely singularity, or irreducible uniqueness.

Every human being, every institution, every firm, every commodity in the world has these four aspects. To reflect this, we might say that every concrete universal is also a concrete singular and its general form will be a quadruple multiplicity. In other words, it can be analysed, at different times, in terms of these four terms. However, we must also remember that there is a transitive aspect of our classification, and therefore we must also ask why we need the classification. All four steps of the foregoing definition of "woman" might be different, for instance, depending on whether I am a genealogical researcher whose objective is to use mitochondrial DNA to trace maternal lineage far back in time, or an events planner whose objective is to make sure that wedding invitations are appropriately addressed according to their gender identity. The concept within empiricist philosophy – that competes with the concept of the concrete universal – is that of the abstract universal. Critical realism suggests that abstract universals do not exist in the world. To the contrary, all universals are concrete (i.e. not abstract). Therefore, any researcher, whether they are concerned primarily with the universal or particular aspects of something, will have to look at these other aspects as well. This has significant implications for interdisciplinarity; in fact, it implies the necessity of interdisciplinarity in research.

Step 4: being as incorporating transformative praxis, that is, human action

This level of the development of ontology deals with transformative agency or praxis. Transformative praxis includes the idea that there is no way that one can "not act"; it is part of our being. Someone may make a decision to *not* do something; and this is an inaction, but it is also a form of action. If they do nothing, the "doing nothing" will issue in inactions of various kinds. It will still be a "doing"; even if it is a "doing" nothing. This is what critical realists call the axiological imperative. Furthermore, in order to do anything, one will have to do something without doing it by doing something else. For instance, one cannot only think about doing it, one also just has to do it. If a writer wants to write something, they cannot do it by thinking about the next sentence that they are going to write: they just have to write it. They may organize their desk, switch off their phone, and set up their computer; but none of this gets the writing done. They may therefore have (ontological, real) transcendental agency – the potential or ability to do something – but this is not the same as, it is not reducible to, the (ontological, real) act or acting itself.

Although one cannot avoid acting, in order to have relevant or directed transformative agency, one needs to satisfy some preconditions. For instance, we need: reasons for our actions; an idea of what it is that we want to achieve and how we aim to achieve it; and it has to be the case that change can occur at all. This sounds like common sense and is something no serious person is likely to deny, but mainstream irrealist philosophy denies this straightforward approach to agency. To put it simply, mainstream philosophy denies that we can arrive at "ought" from "is", which we have already touched on when we explored Hume's (1934/1740) denial that we can arrive at values from facts. In a similar way, mainstream irrealist philosophy also denies that reasons for things are a subset of causes. Hume reflected this denial of agency when he suggested that there is no philosophical reason for him to prefer the scratching of his finger to the destruction of the whole world. Think about this; it means that his actions cannot be guided by the fact that his finger is a much lesser loss than the whole world. At its base, this misunderstanding is the consequence of Hume's denial that there are ontological connections between things. He claimed that all events are entirely loose and separate; it may be that one event follows another, but there is no tie between these events. Hume (1748, Part II) stated that events "seem conjoined but never connected". As such, according to Hume, we have detotalization because things are always atomistic and causation is simply a psychological habit; it is not real. Therefore, irrealism is unable to theorize the concept of intentional causality. We have also already seen that irrealism fails to realize that the category of causality is real or that we have real dispositions or potentials, making the possibility of a concrete utopia non-ontological and therefore not something that can be taken seriously. Furthermore, irrealist philosophy denies the existence of absence, and yet causality is essentially the process of absenting. Therefore, irrealism denies the possibility of agency.

By contrast, critical realism assumes that we can have a constellation of reasons (which form a subset of causes) and that there are emergent powers of the mind (causally efficacious reasons) located in a partially socialized nature in an unsocialized cosmos. Unfortunately, instead of this moral realism and ethical naturalism, in which facts can inform our values, we currently face various problematic, relativist ethical consequences of subjectivist or quasi-objectivist (positivist) irrealism, specifically:

1. Subjective, emotivist moral ideologies for masters, such as the manager, the therapist, the aesthete, the expert, the bureaucrat, the media star, or the soap persona

    This is based on a descriptivist morality that reflects the status quo of actually existing morality. In the transitive dimension it de-moralizes by reflecting (in the intransitive dimension) the morality of an actual, already moralized world. What is ethical is what is normal or usual and failures are assumed to be the result of deviating from the norm.

2. Abstract universalist personalist moral ideologies for slaves

    This ascribes the responsibility for problems to the disconnected individual in an abstract, desocialized, deprocessualized, unmediated way with blame, often followed by punishment (rather than the failure to satisfy needs), as the penalty for failure. This is useful for the masters who can avoid blame and social critique. A good example of this is the way that a husband might blame his wife for "always being the one to start a fight" – but this blame ignores the processes and mediations, most likely the oppression of the woman by her husband, which result in her initiating arguments in an attempt to solve issues and problems (Gunnarsson, 2013). Essentially, it is assumed that the person whose actions are associated with failure is to blame (constant conjunctions indicate causation). Since the masters tend not to carry out the work themselves, the slaves are usually to blame; this serves to deflect critique from the social structures and mechanisms that maintain (and are maintained by) the social hierarchies.

3. Religious or ethnic fundamentalist ethics, accepted on a purely positive basis, i.e. on authority alone

> This displaces the responsibility for determining ethical action onto religious texts or respected people who interpret these texts. In other words, instead of trying to solve problems through social critique, adherents of this position try to solve problems by reiterating a fundamentalist position, often assuming that the root of all problems is a failure to adhere to fundamentalist beliefs.

There are some other implications of the critical realist ontology as it relates to agency. One of these is that, due to holistic causality, and the deep interconnectedness of all being, a change in one part of the world is a fortiori a change in the other. Also, since agents are part of the world, whether they try to address social problems by changing themselves or by changing the world, there is mutuality in both strategies since both result in a change in the world. Another implication of the impossibility of avoiding action is that transformation requires changing (absenting aspects of) what agents are already doing. It requires changes to ourselves and our environment and, if we are to achieve our objectives, there needs to be a balance between our subjective needs and objective possibilities. We also need to be able to trust that the knowledge and analysis that inform our praxis are ultimately based in a moral commitment towards the flourishing of all beings. Furthermore, change involves the multimechanism (interdisciplinary) totality and is therefore also auto-reflexive (reflexivity is the inwardized form of totality). It will also necessarily involve a political transition to a new regime. Given all of these considerations, Bhaskar (2008b/1993: 120, 266) describes praxis as: transformed (autoplastic – changes to self); transformative (alloplastic – changes to the environment); trustworthy; totalizing (all-inclusive and auto-reflexive); transformist (oriented to structural change, informed by explanatory critique and concrete utopianism, and participatory – animating/activating research); and transitional or TTTTTT.

Step 5: being as incorporating reflexivity

This next step is being as agential intentionality, or self-conscious reflexivity. Reflexivity is the ability of an agent or an institution to take account of, monitor, or take stock of their activity; it answers the question: "Are my/our actions faithful to the guiding theory?" Critical realism aims to improve our capacity to be reflexive, or to "walk our talk"; this is the objective of underlabouring. Self-conscious reflexivity results in us taking responsibility for our actions. In order to do this, however, we have to be honest about the reason for our actions. This level is also, in some ways, the level of spirituality, since it relates to the role often played by spirituality in people's lives, namely the role of guiding them to act for "the good" or righteously. It is therefore associated with Bhaskar's so-called spiritual turn (Bhaskar, 2000, 2011, 2012).

As we have seen in the third step of the development of critical realism, reflexivity is basically the inwardized form of totality (Bhaskar, 2008b/1993: 8).

Reflexivity is also auto-reflexive. This is because mismatches between theory and praxis simply are ontological; they are not just subjective or only in the mind. They would exist even if there were no human beings to see them. When these contradictions exist, we may go to great lengths to avoid facing them, but our strategies to avoid facing reflexivity reaffirm its ontological existence.

Psychologically speaking, we can avoid reflexivity – contradictions between our theory and practice – by using the logic of what Jacques Derrida (1998) has called "supplementarity", Sigmund Freud (1923) called "compromise formation", and Festinger and Carlsmith (1959) called cognitive dissonance theory. Essentially, the reflexive process by which these psychological contradictions become self-conscious, that is, the way that a person develops from egocentricity to self-consciousness, is an aspect of the dialectic of self-realization and therefore is in a way a kind of spirituality (Bhaskar, 2016).

Step 6: being as meaningful

Towards the end of the nineteenth century, Friedrich Nietzsche [1844–1900] and Max Weber [1864–1920] argued vigorously that there is no value in the world itself. Supposedly, values are mere projections of human beings onto the world. Similarly, they insisted that there is no meaning in the world in itself. Meaning is supposedly something that human beings project onto the world. This postmodern nihilism led to their fascination with endings. Therefore, the postmoderns talked about:

- the "end of history"
- the end of human beings or man
- the end of the author
- the end of god
- the end of value.

However, contrary to Nietzsche and Weber, we argue that there is meaning in the world. Therefore, the sixth level of ontology is understanding being as meaningful. Critical realism agrees with the primitive view of the world that holds that the world contains valuable or meaningful things and that some (meaningful) things have more value than others; therefore, if a primitive human looked up at the sky and saw a particular cloud, it meant rain, which was valued because then the crops would be watered. In this way, the world was filled with meaningful things, to which values became attached. However, some things are meaningful in a harmful way, such as structural racism, and it would be best to negatively value them and stop reproducing them through our daily actions.

Step 7: being prioritizes identity over difference and unity over split

The seventh step argues for being in terms of the primacy of identity over difference and the primacy of unity over split. The seventh level is interesting because in a way it seems to argue from the opposite viewpoint to the first level. At the first level, we stress the non-identity between things and categories, and the concept of difference is highlighted. However, at the seventh level we assert that, after all, identity is philosophically prior to difference. An example of this might be two people in conversation. Each is totally absorbed in what the other is saying; in this moment, their consciousnesses are in transcendental identification even though their bodies and their beings remain distinct. They are therefore still in the world of duality, even though they have in one way transcended this world – transcended subject/object duality – in their deep conversation. Thus, their consciousnesses are united, yet the sense in which the opposition between subject and object is transcended does not require that we abolish the physical world of duality.

It is also important to note that the sense of identity to which we refer in the seventh step is very different from the punctiform, atomistic identity critiqued in the first stages of the development of critical realism. Rather, it is a differentiated, developing identity, one that changes and moves. It is the sense of identity that one might have when listening to a symphony or admiring a stunningly beautiful sunset. To offer some evidence for the primacy of identity over difference, we can make some non-formal arguments using our ordinary usage of concepts. A basic argument for this step (there are others) is that we cannot say that two things are different unless they have something in common. We cannot say that one person has a different height from another person unless they have something in common, namely height. This suggests the priority of identity over difference, or the priority of unity over split. We could talk loosely about there being several universes, such as the multiple-world argument by Hugh Everett (1956), but basically there can only be one universe because even if there were another universe, there is no way that we can possibly know about it; if there were another universe and it had access to our universe, or it came into contact with our universe, then it would be a part of our universe. For this reason, we talk about the cosmic envelope and we can give it social significance by describing Hegel's (1998/1807) life-and-death struggle. Hegel asked why, when two people (supposedly men) fight a life-and-death struggle, the victor often does not kill the vanquished. He said that this was because it is more important that the victor is able to enjoy the praises of the person he has vanquished than to kill him – he wants someone to say how brave and brilliant he is as a fighter – he wants recognition. However, Ludwig Feuerbach [1804–1872], Karl Marx, and their left-Hegelian successors turned the dialectical tables; they argued that there was another reason why the victor (master) spares the life of the person he vanquishes: he wants to enslave the vanquished, that is, turn him into a servant. However, Marx then argued that eventually the slaves will inherit the world because the master will grow complacent and will be unable to do anything, whereas the slaves will be continually forced to objectify their labour and so begin to see themselves in their products. Eventually, this reaches the point at which the slave is able to overthrow the master and, more importantly, is able to overthrow the master–slave relationship.

The underlying moral of this critical realist dialectic is that when we have a difference, instead of focusing on the difference, it is better to look for the grounds of the difference. Therefore, in terms of, for example, getting on with a neighbour, you both may be very different, but there will be a common ground which unites the difference between you. This has important implications for interdisciplinarity because one of the reasons often given for why disciplinary collaboration fails is that the researchers feel unable to understand or relate to each other. However, we argue here that we can in principle understand or identify with any other human being. This is called *the principle of universal solidarity*.

Note

1 To be fair to Derrida, it seems likely that both critics and advocates of his work have misinterpreted his words "there is nothing beyond the text". Many scholars suggest that this statement was not intended to mean that there is no ontology (Heinze, 2005: 12).

8
CRITICAL REALISM AND THE ALTERNATIVE METATHEORIES/ METHODOLOGIES

Critical realists acknowledge that brilliant and successful science can be done without critical realism, including instances of interdisciplinary work. For instance, many great discoveries have been made using the practices of the experimental natural sciences that arose in the times of Newton and Galileo in the seventeenth century. This is because, despite the inadequacies of mainstream theories of scientific method, mainstream natural science nevertheless has certain relatively adequate practices. These practices exist while at the same time they are not sufficiently theorized. However, although scientists do not have to be critical realists to do good research, they potentially can do even better research, especially in an interdisciplinary context, if they have an improved self-understanding of their successful practice. In this chapter, we argue that critical realism provides science with greater theory/practice consistency compared to alternative methodologies, and that such consistency is greatly enabling of interdisciplinary research. This is an important aspect of the relationship between metatheory and interdisciplinarity since it paves the way for an inclusive and open-minded approach with which to practise interdisciplinary research.

In the social sciences, there is a great deal of ideological contestation around the issue of understanding our research practice. Social scientists interested in a particular social theory or social condition characteristically find that it is coupled to an exciting philosophical position, such as hermeneutics, empiricism, or social constructivism. However, the question then arises as to which of these different philosophical positions is scientific or "proper". For interdisciplinary researchers, the question also arises as to how they can justify using apparently incommensurable methodologies. This is where critical realism is helpful, because it allows scientists to justify their activities from a metatheoretical perspective. However, even if a scientist has a metatheory, this in itself says nothing about the actual method that they might use. This is something that the scientist must work out for themselves in relation to their situation. For example, perhaps a scientist works out that social constructionism applies perfectly in their situation and therefore the only thing that they must analyse is text. This is perfectly acceptable, if the scientist does not rule out the possibility that there are other mechanisms in reality that are not manifest at a textual level.

One of the general advantages of critical realism is that it offers a more inclusive account of ontology and epistemology than any other methodology. Characteristically, as a result of their non-inclusive account of ontology, the alternative methodologies are subject to limitations and conditions that leave them vulnerable to damaging critiques. Roy Bhaskar is not the first writer to point out their weaknesses but his important contribution is that he uses a particularly formidable form of critical analysis, namely immanent critique (cf. Chapter 4).

To begin with, in this chapter, we will look at the strengths and weaknesses of the alternative methodologies. At the end of the chapter, we will consider their rational place within a more comprehensive account that critical realism tends to describe. Specifically, we will discuss critical realism's advantages over:

- empiricism;
- neo-Kantianism;
- hermeneutics; and
- social-constructivism.

Empiricism

Empiricism is the oldest methodology in the field. In terms of its simplest definition, empiricism makes use of the Humean formula for universality, which is that a scientific law is a constant conjunction of more or less atomistic events. The problem with only looking for empirical regularities is that these are neither necessary nor sufficient for a causal law. Contrary to what scientists might claim, their empirical work is the process by which they discover or uncover structures and mechanisms (or transfactuals) that operate in a law-like way at the level of the real, and not necessarily at the level of the actual. Transfactuals play out in the following ways.

Scenario 1: The transfactual *is not manifest* in a particular sequence of events, as it plays out in an *open-system* context; yet even when the mechanism it describes is not manifest in such a sequence of events, the law still operates. For example, prior to 1968 in the UK, if a rhesus-negative mother had a rhesus-positive baby, her next rhesus-positive baby, due to the mechanisms of her immune system, was at risk of oxygen deprivation due to haemolytic disease. However, these days this problem is prevented because of medical interventions. There is no longer an empirical regularity between rhesus-negative mothers and oxygen-deprived babies in the UK. However, this does not mean that the causal law (mechanism of her immune system) ceases to exist in Western countries: it is still real, even if it is not actualized. Therefore, the Humean formula cannot be necessary for a scientific law.

Scenario 2: The transfactual *is manifest in a qualified way*, as it plays out in an *open-system* context; this is because it is actualized in combination with the workings of a great many other mechanisms, and this results in an imperfect sequence of events related to the transfactual. Therefore, although Western countries have effectively removed the correlation between rhesus-negative mothers and oxygen-deprived babies, this is not necessarily the case in countries with poor health care. Furthermore, the babies of some rhesus-negative mothers will not be affected in the rare event that the father is also rhesus negative.

Scenario 3: The transfactual *perfectly manifests* in a particular conjunction of events, as it plays out in a *closed-system* context artificially achieved by isolating variables in a laboratory.

The only scenario that empiricism truly describes is scenario 3, and since this is often technically and/or ethically impossible to achieve in the social sciences, it seems odd that empiricism remains the methodology of choice for social policy-makers. Empiricism theorizes the empirical invariance measured in scientific laboratory practices, but it does not provide a theory that includes all the conditions that are needed for the empirical invariance. Empiricism therefore starts at – limits itself to – the laboratory situation whereas critical realism moves outside the laboratory situation and asks what conditions are necessary to establish the empirical invariance and why it is necessary to establish it.

However, the empiricists' faith in correlations as the only evidence of causation also leads to other problems. For instance, it is possible to have an empirical correlation that is purely accidental or circumstantial, but that plays out because of the operation of a number of causally unrelated mechanisms. For example, there may be a perfect positive correlation between the amount of red wine that people drink and how long they live. However, in reality there may be nothing to connect the two; and therefore the correlation is purely accidental. Alternatively, perhaps the correlation is circumstantial. Therefore, the correlation exists not because wine increases longevity, but because people who drink red wine are more likely to be from a higher socio-economic bracket, and have better access to health care; thus the correlation does not provide information about the effect of wine on human beings. Consequently, drinking a glass of red wine a day may not help a person to live longer unless there is a causal mechanism for the red wine to improve longevity. Trained scientists, and many well-informed laypeople, acknowledge that "correlations do not equal causation". However, the contradiction lies in the way that, despite this acknowledgement, scientists continue to focus their research efforts on finding correlations rather than transfactuals. Statistical correlations remain the socially sanctioned way to arrive at "evidence-based" research to inform public policy. The excessive trust placed in correlations is the result of empiricist universalism, which leaves researchers no alternative. In the absence of the idea of transfactuals, it is assumed that policy made on the basis of correlations is the better of two evils: the alternative evil being policy based on ideology, hearsay, or even superstition.

Ironically, the fact that the scientists are successful (carry out the axiological necessities of epistemology) while nevertheless their philosophy of science fails to reflect what they actually do, protects their philosophy from collapsing. This mismatch between what the scientists say that they are doing and what they are actually doing is an example of a TINA formation, discussed earlier (cf. Chapter 7). Specifically, scientists argue that knowledge gained from inside the laboratory is worth much more than knowledge from outside the laboratory. Nevertheless, contradictorily, they also want their results to be applied to the open-systemic world. Therefore, they act as if the laws of nature that they discover are transfactual, that is, that they operate outside laboratory conditions; and they act as if they can discover these laws that operate outside laboratory conditions.

This critique of empiricism is well-established and many philosophers of science have long recognized that constant conjunctions of atomistic events are neither necessary nor sufficient for establishing causal laws. These philosophers have theorized that it is necessary to talk about "something more" or a surplus element, as well as constant conjunctions. Some of these philosophers, namely the neo-Kantians, identified a surplus element in terms of Kant's categories, or models. They said that, in addition to a constant conjunction of events or empirical regularity, we also need a good model to allow us to make sense of reality. This is an important step and we will look at this in more detail in the next section.

Neo-Kantianism

Kant talked very strictly about the operation of categories which he thought were necessary for the intelligibility of empirical experience. The philosophers that we call the neo-Kantians adopt a more catholic view of what it is that you need to add to the empirical invariance. They agree with Kant that you have the empirical invariance and "something more" but they are not so strict about what the "something more" is. The neo-Kantians Mary Hesse [1924–2016] and Rom Harré [1927–] are in many respects fairly close to critical realism. They argued for the importance of models. Similarly, Stephen Toulmin [1922–2009] and Norwood Hanson [1924–1967] argued that, in addition to empirical regularities, it was also necessary to have a good metaphor. However, they did not have an explicitly stratified ontology and therefore they lacked a plausible rationale for these models or "surplus elements" to be about something real and in the world; instead they located the models in the scientific mind or community. Furthermore, since their models were not about something real, they could not choose between better or worse models as it was not possible to test the models or metaphors against independent reality. Critical realism improves on their position with its concepts of (a) ontological realism, where the model refers to structures and mechanisms at the level of the real in a stratified ontology; and (b) judgemental rationality, which is the process by which a researcher can decide between competing theories or models. Using the process of judgemental rationality, a researcher is able to choose the most plausible surplus element or model that best explains the currently available evidence. For critical realists, contra the neo-Kantians, a model identifies a stratum of reality; it is not merely something in the researcher's head.

The mistake that is made by both the empiricists and neo-Kantians alike is that empirical regularities are assumed to be necessary for causal laws or scientific statements to be established. This mistake is associated with a nexus of philosophical problems, the most well-known being the problem of induction. The problem of induction can be described as follows: even if a person has only ever seen white swans, they cannot claim that therefore all swans are white, because it is always possible that a black swan will turn up. This is exactly what happened historically. Europeans thought that all swans were white because they had only ever seen white swans, but then they went to South America and discovered that there were also black swans. This was a devastating indictment against induction. The problem of induction is that, if the evidence for a scientific law consists only of instances, then it can never actually be confirmed because no matter how many instances exist to satisfy the causal law, or the law-like statement, it will always be possible for a counter-instance to turn up. Some philosophers such as Karl Popper (2014/1963) tried to get around the problem of induction by suggesting that, while it is not possible to confirm a law-like state, it is possible to falsify it. However, the falsification argument does not stand for three reasons:

1. Given the open-system nature of the world, most law-like statements, if interpreted empirically, are eventually falsified due to mediating factors. A statement can be either empirical or universal but not both.
2. It is never sufficient for a single instance of a falsification to count because the falsification must be repeatable and in general universalizable. This returns us back to the original problem of induction and the lack of warrant for the supposition of the uniformity of nature.
3. The response to a supposedly falsifying instance is usually to modify the statement or theory rather than to reject it completely; thus the law that all swans are white is qualified to include the claim that some swans are black, but one day perhaps brown swans will be seen.

The critical realist solution of the problem of induction is to say that we can rationally believe, for instance, that all emeralds are green – not because we only have instances of green emeralds, but because we have a theory that explains why emeralds are green. Emeralds are green because of their particular chemical make-up; indeed, emeralds cannot be anything other than green. Rubies and emeralds are similar in chemical composition, except that emeralds also contain beryl. Remove the beryl, and emeralds would be red rubies. This theory for why emeralds are green describes a higher level of reality. In virtue of this higher level of reality, it is not possible for something that satisfies the criteria of being an emerald to be anything other than green. Therefore, the resolution of the problem of induction lies in this higher level of reality that implies ontological structure, or depth.

To explain further, scientists do not restrict their activities to accumulating or generating instances or empirical invariances and trying to refute correlations.

Rather, the whole point of the scientific enterprise is to build an understanding of the deeper, most likely interdisciplinary, generative mechanisms or causal structures that are at work to produce empirical instances and correlations. This is what science is all about. Science is not about collecting information about our existing level of reality; it is about uncovering the causes of it, and this means going deeper into it, or more fully into it. The real problem with empiricism, which also applies to neo-Kantianism, is the actualist assumption that everything in life is actual. This is not true; there is a domain of reality that is not manifest in actual events or empirical objects. In this deeper domain of reality, things cannot be sensed empirically; we must surmise their existence from the available evidence. Once it is clear that reality is ontologically structured in this manner, then the problem of induction falls away.

Furthermore, the empiricist version of science is rather dull because it is only about describing the world. However, the beauty of science is that it allows us to uncover something more about the natural sciences and about nature, namely the structure behind the patterns of events generating it. It allows us to uncover things that we do not yet know about ourselves and our societies, and our interactions with nature. Both Kantianism and empiricism presuppose the level of the empirical. Nevertheless, while empiricism insists that the world consists of only empirical regularities, Kantianism says there is something more to knowledge. That "something more" is structure. The problem with Kantianism is that the structure is presumed to exist only at the level of the transitive dimension; its version of structure is only epistemological. Its theory of models (of structure) would be fine if it acknowledged that there is a reality that the models are trying to capture, a reality constituted by mechanisms and structures. This is the difference between a neo-Kantian approach and a scientific or critical realist approach. The latter admits that the models are about something real.

Kantians struggle to reconcile their approach with the way that models or categories are epistemically relative, i.e. socially produced and socially changeable. This is not a problem for critical realists since we can use the available evidence to choose between the different versions of the models. However, since Kantian models are supposedly not about anything real, they tend towards being relativist; in other words, it is difficult to find evidence one way or another for the truth of any particular claim. The strength of empiricism – what it is really good at – is its ability to describe empirical procedures and to carry out empirical testing. However, it is not good at describing what the rationale is for these procedures; for that the empiricist scientist needs a concept of ontological structure and depth. The strength of neo-Kantianism is that it demonstrates the necessity for the scientific mind or scientific imagination. It shows the necessity for us to acknowledge that science is more than just accumulating data. That "something more" is what we imaginatively construct. However, the whole point of that "something more" is to identify the real, causal structures or generative mechanisms (which are usually interdisciplinary). And these causal structures are themselves the products of deeper and wider structures.

Hermeneutics

In the field of social science, empiricism is implausible as it is strictly stated – although this does not mean as it is practised. It is implausible because there are no universal generalizations in the open system of society of the type that empiricism requires. As a result some methodologists – the hermeneuticists – suggest that there is a huge gulf between the natural and the human worlds. For the hermeneuticists: (a) the natural world is general and repeatable, while the human world is unique or idiosyncratic; and (b) the human world is linguistic or meaningful in a way that the natural world is not. The hermeneuticists were partly right. Just as empiricism has its truth that experience is an important aspect of epistemology and neo-Kantianism has its truth that we need to build models, so too does hermeneutics have its truth. This truth is that both the social sciences and the human sciences are hermeneutical, that is to say, they are linguistic and conceptualized. However, this doesn't mean that everything in social life is just language and it doesn't mean that conceptuality exhausts society. While it is true that social life is linguistic, we cannot then conclude that social life exists only in language. Instead, it is better to say that social activity is *concept-dependent*, but not *concept-exhausted*. Therefore, while we have a concept of *hunger*, this concept is not the end of the story; the physical lack of food is also important. Furthermore, this means that our particular conceptualizations are both corrigible and subject to critique, and that there may be dimensions of the social that have not been conceptualized. The hermeneuticists, to the contrary, assumed that people's conceptualizations were incorrigible, that is, that they were the whole story and that they could not be critiqued. Also, the hermeneuticists did not embark on interdisciplinary research because they did not acknowledge that humans are materially embodied as well as conceptualizing beings; they therefore had no reason to measure and count the material features of society. They only wanted to record and interpret our conceptual activity. The corrigibility of our conceptualizations is the basis for the scepticism of the so-called "masters" of suspicion, such as Kant, Hegel, and Marx, and more recently Nietzsche and Freud. They were all concerned to critique illusion in the human world.

Social constructionism

Social constructionism combines neo-Kantianism with hermeneutics. It therefore takes the Kantian position – that in science, or in a disciplinary study of a subject matter, one cannot avoid interpretation – and combines it with the hermeneutic idea that social life is linguistic in character. Some critical realists (such as Andrew Sayer, 2000: 90) suggest that social constructionism comes in two forms: weak and strong. Weak social constructionism acknowledges both the transitive and intransitive aspects of reality. It is the idea that intransitive social reality always comes with its transitive interpretation and it is consistent with critical realism. Strong social constructionism insists that the interpretation is all that there is, that social reality just is language – it is "language all the way down". In this book, when we refer to social constructionism, we refer to the strong version. Such a position is morally irresponsible and outrageous. This is because there are serious problems that affect humanity and these problems need to be understood in an interdisciplinary way; it is vital to be able to describe them, to theorize them, and to critique them. Yet, social constructionism disallows this critique. However, strong social constructionism is easily refuted. For instance, social constructionists collect their salaries. They go home, stop at the supermarket, and buy various things to eat for dinner like everyone else. If they have a toothache, they go to the dentist. They don't just change their vocabulary; and, therefore, there is a part of their practice that they do not theorize. Consequently, social constructionists are subject to TINA formations, just like Hume. And like Hume, they become notorious and famous by saying increasingly outrageous things. Unfortunately, many people believe them and act on the outrageous suggestions. Hume was in many respects an academic hero. He was a very likeable character. However, ultimately his work led to the idea that everything is acceptable – anything goes – and that our values have no basis in reality. The consequence of his scholarship was that the possibility of critique was denied. Hume was a smart, complacent, eighteenth-century gentleman who was doing very well and it seems plausible that the motive behind his position was that he did not want to upset the status quo. Perhaps this same motive explains why social constructionism is so popular today. Perhaps this claim is arguable, but the important point is that social constructionism is profoundly wrong.

Critical realism is anti-imperialist

Nevertheless, the criticism of strong social constructionism does not mean that there is no value in the work of such postmodernist thinkers as Derrida or Foucault. To the contrary, these are extremely suggestive writers and we certainly advocate the study of them. It merely means that, if we use their ideas, we should balance our analysis with the acknowledgement that there is an extra-discursive reality. The criticism of strong social constructionism also does not mean that the examination of discourse, text, and documents is irrelevant. To the contrary, such analysis is essential to social science and indeed hermeneutics is a necessary starting point of social science. Critical realism therefore embraces the alternative methodologies and agrees that language and text are very important, as are the writings of Hume and Foucault. What critical realism questions is the imperialism of these alternative methodologies. The imperialism of empiricism insists that science must only be about numbers and statistics. The imperialism of neo-Kantianism insists that while we have numbers and can devise models around them, we must not try to say that these models reflect or correspond to reality in any way. The imperialism of the language-oriented social constructionists insists that there is nothing more to social science than interpretation. Critical realism's anti-imperialist stance is profoundly enabling of interdisciplinarity.

As social scientists, our objective is therefore to give an account of the world that includes instances such as empirical regularities, but that also includes non-regularities. Once we come out of the Humean straitjacket, we can look at empirical regularities in a looser way, a way that is empirically suggestive but nevertheless scientifically proper. Most importantly, our approach will include structures and (interdisciplinary) generative mechanisms. Reality has a depth to it and it is that depth that we are trying to uncover. We want to achieve a more inclusive account of reality and therefore it may be necessary to mesh together different branches of sociology, and even other disciplines, in interdisciplinary research. If we allow that certain beliefs might be superficial or illusory, then we will be motivated to look more deeply at them. If we find that the beliefs are indeed mistaken, we can then explore how the discourses or texts that reflect these beliefs function as causally efficacious absences. Even if a belief is not true, if a person acts on it, then it is a causally efficacious bit of reality. The terrible thing is that people act on illusions; for instance most wars, perhaps all wars, are based on such illusions.

One of the consequences of the dominance of the irrealist metatheoretical positions hitherto is that we talk about "interdisciplinarity". This is an epistemologically based term that refers to many disciplines. Ideally, it should be possible to talk in an ontological mode and refer instead to something along the lines of "intermeshing of mechanisms" or "mechanismicity". However, because ontology has been taboo in Western science or in Western philosophy, we do not have a convenient word for "intermeshing of mechanisms". Therefore, the very language of interdisciplinarity is somewhat mystifying.

Critical realism is epistemologically all-inclusive

Epistemologically, critical realism is more inclusive than the other metatheories as it demonstrates both why we need statistics and why we need to look at discourse, and it fits these different approaches into a more comprehensive account of the scientific process. While other metatheories focus on one specific area of investigation, critical realism tries to give a picture of the whole, including the insights from other metatheories. This is called the *critical realist embrace*. It is intrinsically supportive of interdisciplinarity. It acknowledges the importance of (a) the descriptive moment in the natural sciences, which is the moment associated with measuring things and carrying out experiments; (b) the neo-Kantian moment, which is the retroductive moment associated with the identification of a generative structure; (c) the point at which we must eliminate alternative theories; and then (d) the point at which we come back to an empirical moment. This all-inclusivity is what makes interdisciplinarity possible and the alternative metatheories were not able to support interdisciplinarity in this way because they left out important aspects of ontology.

This brings us to the end of Part II. We now move to Part III, where we try to apply the principles of critical realism and interdisciplinarity to certain practical aspects of wellbeing.

PART III
Applied interdisciplinary research

We have allowed the bio-psycho-social model to become the bio-bio-bio model.
Steven Sharfstein (2005: 2045)
President of the American Psychiatric Association

9
BIOPHYSICAL INTERVENTIONS ARE NOT ENOUGH

The hidden (holistic) healing ensemble

If the physical levels of reality are closed, that is, if they essentially determine the genesis of wellbeing (or lack of wellbeing, such as health disorders and psychological dysfunction), then there would be no need to look at mechanisms at the other levels and how they interact; there would be no need for interdisciplinarity. However, there is evidence that the physical levels of reality are not closed and therefore factors at other levels, such as those of a psychological and social nature, are significant in explaining the absence of wellbeing. For instance, we know that long working hours increase the chance of cardiovascular disease and that loneliness detrimentally affects the functioning of the immune system (Kivimäki et al., 2015; Cole et al., 2015). Some researchers suggest that 75% of visits to the doctor are stress-related (Ninabahen et al., 2011).

This leads us to reflect on those aspects of health care that are often ignored because they are extra to the biophysical, which we call the *hidden (holistic) healing ensemble*, and which we will discuss later in this chapter. However, we will begin by exploring one of the most compelling pieces of evidence that health issues are not purely understandable in terms of their biophysical causality: the well-documented phenomenon of the placebo effect.

The placebo effect described

The placebo effect was first described by anaesthesiologist Henry K. Beecher [1904–1976]. In the usual scenario, a placebo – an imitation treatment, such as sugar, saline solution, or even distilled water – is given to a patient and about 35% of the time they will experience an improvement in their condition (Beecher, 1955). The effect is not limited to helpful changes. If a patient expects to experience side-effects of the treatment, such as nausea or stomach complaints, these can also become manifest. This is known as the nocebo effect (Benedetti et al., 2007).

However, research has further demonstrated that regardless of whether the patient is receiving a placebo, how much time and care the physician devotes to a patient is also correlated to a positive clinical outcome. Finniss et al. (2010: 686) state:

> Recent research demonstrates that placebo effects are genuine psychobiological events attributable to the overall therapeutic context, and that these effects can be robust in both laboratory and clinical settings. There is also evidence that placebo effects can exist in clinical practice, even if no placebo is given.

How does the placebo effect work?

The exact mechanism for how the placebo effect works is unknown (Benedetti et al., 2005). However, in terms of reducing pain, it seems that opioid and/or non-opioid mechanisms are involved via expectations and/or conditioning mechanisms in the context of the placebo administration (the psycho-social-physical environment). Benedetti et al. also demonstrate that while expectation is a key in pain-related placebo effects, this is not the case in hormone-related placebo effects, which require conditioning instead; for instance, when previous experience of the efficacy of a treatment is followed by a treatment that looks the same but is merely an inactive substance, this results in a placebo effect even if the patients are told not to expect positive results.

A theory of the placebo effect as ergonic efficiency

A possible explanation for the placebo effect is the well-acknowledged tendency for systems to maximize energy efficiency (Odum, 1994). Bhaskar (2008b/1993: 120) has suggested that ergonic (energy) efficiency is a key aspect of action aimed at human wellbeing. In human systems, the study of such efficiency has been called ergonomics. That the human body has a limited amount of energy/resources and must therefore restrict usage in one area to compensate for increased usage in another area, is demonstrated by the way that the body sends blood away from the skeletal muscles, to the intestines, after a meal (Chou, 1983). In terms of explaining the placebo effect, if someone is in pain, first they must escape (fight or flee) the source of the pain. There is no point in putting resources into the healing process if the source of the danger is not escaped first. Once the organism has found safety, it no longer needs to be motivated by pain; neither does it need high levels of adrenalin or other stress-related hormones. By reducing these things, it can transfer its resources towards the immune system and the body's inbuilt healing processes. The receipt of medicine – or simply being in a safe environment and surrounded by trusted people – may be a signal to the person's body that safety is at hand and that they are going to be taken care of. Thus, the pain, which has served its purpose of getting the person the help that they need, can be reduced along with fight or flee hormones. It seems plausible that this results in the placebo effect, especially if the medication (placebo) is supposed to reduce pain. In the case of non-pain-related medical issues, where conditioning rather than expectation is the key to the placebo effect, it makes sense that once a person learns that a certain intervention is going to help, then initially they will need the skills associated with "fight or flee" hormones, such as hyper-vigilance and perhaps strength, to find or make ready that intervention. Once the intervention is at hand, it may be useful to switch off the "fight or flee" response even before administering the intervention to ensure its optimal functioning. In this way, more resources are sent to the immune system and it can begin to carry out its healing action. In theory, this decrease in the "fight or flee" bodily state may result in health improvements, even if the intervention is merely a placebo, simply because the body now has more access to resources for its innate healing processes to become fully functional.

That humans can subconsciously switch on or off their immune and pain responses is well-established. For instance, evidence that humans can subconsciously switch on their immune responses in the absence of actual antigens is demonstrated by research on asthma. In one study, asthma suffers were asked to inhale a non-irritating odorant. This odorant was labelled either "asthmogenic" or "therapeutic". The level of nitric oxide in the participants' exhaled air – a marker of airway inflammation – was then measured. It remained unchanged in the group who thought that the smell was therapeutic, but it immediately and significantly began to increase in the group who thought that it was asthmogenic (Rodriguez, 2015). In some contexts, such a reaction may be useful, as it readies the body to face allergens before it encounters them. Evidence that humans can subconsciously switch off their pain is provided by the use of hypnosis as pain relief, which has been reported in a number of studies (Cyna, McAuliffe and Andrew, 2004). Such evidence, along with other evidence such as the negative effect that stress and loneliness have on wellbeing, contradicts a purely body-based, linear cause-and-effect understanding of pain and allergenic reactions.

It therefore seems safe to conclude that to fully address issues of health and wellbeing, not only the physical and biological, but also the psycho-social aspects of disease need to be considered. This commits the health professional to, in principle, the conception of a radically holistic and laminated approach to his or her own activity, set within the wider policy context which is, in turn, set within the wider society. Addressing issues of health and wellbeing in such a way results in considering what we have called the hidden (holistic) healing ensemble.

The hidden (holistic) healing ensemble

The paradox of complementary medicine is that it is surprisingly successful and popular despite the frequent absence of a scientifically accepted understanding of how it works. However, the existence of multiple causal mechanisms may help us to explain this paradox because complementary medicine may attend to certain, usually hidden mechanisms. We call these mechanisms the *hidden (holistic) healing ensemble* and they include, for example:

- human interaction, such as touch and empathy;
- fully understanding the intention and mechanism of the intervention;
- avoiding negative suggestions (such as avoiding Googling the symptoms);
- length of time spent with the health consultant;
- degree to which the patient has confidence in the health and wellbeing interventions;
- the effect of the surroundings on the patients' psychological state of being;
- amount of attention provided; and
- other parts of the patient's life (problems with their job, relationship, debt, etc.).

These factors play a significant role in the complementary context, but they are often seen as an optional extra and, perhaps due to increasing financial (managerial) constraints, they are often left out of a standard biomedical approach. The degree to which the hidden healing ensemble is undervalued differs between countries. For example, it is noticeably absent from highly managerialized medical contexts such as in the UK and USA; but in Belgium and Switzerland it is relatively accepted that a comprehensive battery of measures and policies is necessary to deal with health disorders (World Health Organization, 2013: 64). It is perhaps ironic that measures implemented to save money may do the opposite. For example, several studies have shown that when complementary therapies are used for podalic malposition and labour pain there are significant reductions in costs; some estimate savings of hundreds of Euros per patient (World Health Organization, 2013: 64; van den Berg et al., 2010; Manyande and Grabowska, 2009).

In the next chapter, we will consider in more detail how a critical realist conception of interdisciplinarity can guide health and wellbeing professionals at each stage of the medical programme, from initially deciding on whether or not a disease exists, to finding a cure and healing it. We consider this process to include seven key stages, which we call the seven enigmas of healing.

10
THE SEVEN ENIGMAS OF HEALING

In the introduction, we mentioned that two functions define contemporary medicine: a scientific function, aimed at understanding deep, explanatory causality; and a healing function, aimed at achieving the well-functionality of the human being-in-activity in his or her natural and social context and modelled in terms of four-planar social being (cf. Chapter 5). The scientific function involves absenting our lack of knowledge about an issue, moving to greater completeness in our understanding; while the healing function involves absenting the lack of health and wellbeing, that is, removing (or at least alleviating) causes and symptoms, resulting in the fullest expression possible of wellbeing for any particular individual.

In this chapter, we explore the implications of these two functions in terms of what we call the seven enigmas of healing and we illustrate them by reference to: electromagnetic hypersensitivity, the Diagnostic and Statistical Manual of Mental Disorders (DSM), diabetes, Acquired Immune Deficiency Disorder (AIDS), Alzheimer's disease, coronary heart disease, and anorexia nervosa, among others. The "seven enigmas" facing the health practitioner are:

1. *What is it?* (the enigma of diagnosis);
2. *What are its signs and symptoms?* (the enigma of symptomology);
3. *What causes it?* (the enigma of causation);
4. *What will/would cure it or alleviate it?* (the enigma of healing);
5. *What would have prevented it?* (the enigma of prevention);
6. *How is it experienced?* (the enigma of interpretation);
7. *How are we to cure and alleviate it?* (the enigma of intervention/treatment/therapy/rehabilitation).

The first five enigmas relate to the scientific function of medicine (discovery); and the last two relate to its healing function (application), although it should be noted that these two functions are closely interrelated, and therefore this is consistent with the "theorem of the contingent duality and simultaneity of discovery and application" (cf. Chapter 6). Notice that the term "cure or alleviate" occurs in two of the enigmas. This is because there is a difference between knowing, transfactually, *what* would cure or alleviate something and knowing *how* to apply this transfactual universal in the actual/empirical mediated context of a particular patient. Recall that a statement – in this case a statement about curing or alleviating – can be either universal or actual/empirical but not both (cf. Chapter 7). This is because of the open system and the impossibility of regular constant conjunctions of events. It means that there cannot be a one-to-one relationship between the universal scientific and actual/empirical healing functions.

The first enigma: What is it?

We must answer this question in terms of the two dimensions of reality; namely the intransitive and transitive dimensions (cf. Chapter 2). When we ask the question "What is it?" from the perspective of the intransitive dimension, this relates to the ontological status of "it"; that is, does "it" actually exist and what is its nature? It is not always possible to easily determine the ontological status of something. At the level of the real, we can only know whether something exists based on its effects. This can present challenges to the medical practitioner as it may not be possible to measure the thing itself directly. This is one reason that we can consider this question to be enigmatic. Furthermore, since there is no one-to-one correspondence between "it" as the referent and the words that we use to represent "it", or the readings from the instruments used to measure "it", there is always a chance that some further piece of evidence might surface to change how we define a health issue.

Does electromagnetic hypersensitivity exist?

An example is to be found in the debate over whether or not electromagnetic hypersensitivity exists. As wireless telecommunication continues to proliferate, health professionals are more frequently faced with patients presenting symptoms that they claim are connected with exposure to electromagnetic radiation (EMR):

> Some scientists and clinicians acknowledge the phenomenon of hypersensitivity to EMR resulting from common exposures such as wireless systems and electrical devices in the home or workplace; others suggest that electromagnetic hypersensitivity (EHS) is psychosomatic or fictitious.
>
> *(Genius and Lipp, 2012: 103)*

Electromagnetic hypersensitivity certainly exists on the surface, i.e. it exists in the sense that you can really see the symptoms, such as headache, fatigue, stress, sleep disturbances, burning sensations, and rashes, among others. But is electricity, via some kind of unknown mechanism, the cause of these symptoms? Or, is there something else involved which mediates the two, and makes them appear connected, for example, does electrical equipment such as fluorescent lights and automatic doors produce high-frequency sounds that affect the health of humans? Thus, the problem may not be the electricity per se but rather the sound produced by the machines using the electricity (Leighton, 2016). People who suffer from electromagnetic hypersensitivity say that they are sensitive to very small amounts of electrical energy. However, several blind experiments have failed to show that there is a connection and such people are unable to identify when they are or are not being subjected to these low levels of electromagnetism (Röösli, 2008). Nevertheless, when sufferers move into specially equipped dwellings that keep out exposure to electricity, they no longer show the symptoms in question. This raises the general problem of how electromagnetic fields can affect the biological system and whether or not this may be an example of the nocebo effect, which is similar to the placebo effect, but negative symptoms are expected and thus experienced (Rubin et al., 2006). For now, it seems that there is simply not enough evidence to conclusively agree on whether or not electromagnetic hypersensitivity actually exists.

When we consider the question, "What is it?" from the perspective of the transitive dimension, we need to look at the purpose behind the question, or the objective of our research. In Chapter 4, we mentioned that we cannot answer the question of how many students are in a room until we know why we are asking the question. Is it for setting out the tea cups? If this is the case, then we should not include the student on the other side of the phone. Or is it to deliver handouts? If this is the case, then we should include the student present at the other end of the phone. Similarly, in terms of health and wellbeing issues, we need to understand the social context of the issue when we ask the question, "What is it?" Therefore, we will answer the question, "What is diabetes?" differently depending on our objectives. For example, the question must be answered differently depending on whether we are trying to ensure regional supplies of insulin and therefore need to look at the epidemiology of diabetes, or we are trying to work out the best way to treat people with diabetes, and therefore need to know such details as dosages appropriate to body weight.

Also related to the question of "What is it?" at the level of the transitive dimension is the question of classification and the reason for labelling people. If we want to take care of a person who has a particular health issue, it is necessary both to identify the issue, and to link it with the person. For instance, if a person uses a wheelchair and needs a hotel room with disabled facilities, they need to identify themselves as having certain disabilities. In this case, names and labels are useful, even necessary, to allow people with disabilities to fully participate in social life. Similarly, if a certain group of people is suffering from discrimination and we aim to advocate for their fair treatment, we also need to label them. Unfortunately, such names and labels are also necessary in order to oppress people. Because labels can be used to discriminate against people, many people prefer not to be labelled at all. If we consider the issue of HIV, many sufferers prefer to keep their HIV status a secret. This can cause them other problems, because friends and family may be mistrustful or unsupportive over what may seem like inexplicable and unnecessary changes in diet and other secretive behaviour (secretly taking pills and going to the doctor). However, even those people who are "out" about their status are often highly sensitive about how they are labelled. For instance, over the past several decades of the HIV/AIDS epidemic, the labels applied to people suffering from AIDS have included (Fordham, 2014: 49): in the early 1990s, PWA (people with AIDS); this later transformed to PLWA (people living with AIDS); and then to PLWHA (people living with HIV/AIDS). Some of these changes reflect greater understanding of the biophysical nature of the disease; others reflect the need to change stereotyped social perceptions. In a world where discrimination against people affected by AIDS really exists, there will always be a tension in the labelling process between the advantages of receiving appropriate care for one's condition, and the disadvantages of being singled out for oppression. Being sensitive to the way that a person with a health problem prefers to describe their condition is a way to demonstrate one's commitment to using the label to assist them rather than to harm them. It also demonstrates an understanding of the need to have an interdisciplinary understanding of the disease, since the way that we describe a person suffering from a disease has social and economic implications (McPherson and Armstrong, 2006). Significantly, when labels are to be used to oppress, they are often exaggerated to the point of stereotyping because people have so much to gain or lose by how they are labelled (Bowker and Star, 2000). The potential for labels to be used to oppress motivated postmodernists to be suspicious of labels altogether and to call them acts of violence (Derrida, 1998). There is no need to go as far as the postmodernists, who tried to avoid labelling altogether, but it is important to recognize the great power given to us by labels, and the need to use this power responsibly.

The curious case of drapetomania

Although a great deal of variability is allowed by epistemological relativism, this variability is not unlimited and we are prevented from falling into the trap of "anything goes" by ontological realism. Let us consider the curious phenomenon of drapetomania. This "disease" was invented by Samuel Cartwright, an American physician, in 1851 to explain the fact that slaves were running away. From Cartwright's perspective, the runaway slaves were mad, or at least pathologically irrational, because they were exchanging a secure plantation environment – that provided food, lodging, and at least some basic education – for a jeopardous existence. Of course, from the slaves' perspective, they were escaping an inhuman social order erected on the denial of something essential to human beings: their freedom. How do we decide which perspective is correct? We can reject the claim that the runaway slaves were mad and prefer the idea that they were sane, because the latter explanation takes into account more of the situation/evidence (it takes into account the human need for freedom, which Cartwright's perspective ignores). Similarly, if a pamphlet on diabetes sponsored by a pharmaceutical company strategically leaves out important information, we can argue that its presentation of the facts is inadequate by pointing out the missing information.

The second enigma: What are its signs and symptoms?

Signs and symptoms are present at the empirical level of reality, since we can experience and measure them. Ontologically speaking, signs and symptoms therefore represent only a small part of reality, and merely indicate towards the deeper reality, which we can only know about through transfactuals. Nevertheless, signs and symptoms are the primary way for us to draw conclusions about "what is". Commonly, health and wellbeing practitioners commit the *epistemic fallacy*, in that they confuse their empirical measurements for the disease itself. This is problematic because it can give a false sense of confidence – reducing the process of diagnosis to the simple ticking of boxes. This can blind practitioners to the truth of a situation because, in the open-system world, a disease-causing structure or mechanism present at the level of the real may not exhibit itself in a typical way, due to other factors. Alternatively, similar symptoms may be the manifestation of different diseases. In other words, there is often a mismatch between symptoms and diseases (see Chapter 5 for the way that trends and mechanisms play out in open systems).

A consequence of the epistemic fallacy, in which measures of reality are assumed to be the reality itself (often called reification), is that we may fail to identify the signs and symptoms until the onset of the disease is too far advanced to take any effective action. This is particularly true of certain kinds of cancers. Late diagnosis of cancer reduces the chance of recovery. To prevent this mistake, it may be that we need to cast the net wider to identify symptoms; we should avoid relying on a set of "boxes" of diagnostic symptoms to "tick" (although such boxes may be a good starting point). Although false positives due to "casting the net wider" are a genuine and legitimate concern – because of the waste of resources and the unnecessary subjection of the patient to uncomfortable procedures, such as biopsies – there is nevertheless little evidence that programmes that incentivize narrow, tick-box behaviour among general practitioners, such as the UK's Quality and Outcomes Framework (QOF), are beneficial (Ryan et al., 2016; Roland and Guthrie, 2016). Perhaps we can overcome some of our hesitation to act when there seems to be some reason to do so, but not enough boxes are ticked, if we trust a critical realist research methodology that includes: the search for, and the obtaining of, absent information (broad-based empirical descriptive research, led by the need to absent absences, in order to get a full picture of the situation); the judicious application of already existing theory (retrodiction); and judgemental rationality (elimination of inadequate competing theories). In this way, if the official boxes are not adequately ticked, but cancer is the best explanation for those boxes that *are* ticked, and perhaps others not in the official list, then there is a good argument that we should proceed under the assumption that it may be cancer. If we cannot decide between two competing explanations (for example, the symptoms could be due to cancer *or* indigestion), then the critical realist commitment to absenting absent knowledge would require further tests to gain the information required to make a rational judgement between the two. In an ideal world, the diagnostic success of a medical practitioner would not be judged according to whether they had "ticked the boxes" of empirical evidence, but whether their diagnosis demonstrated explanatory power – the ability to adequately explain the evidence compared to competing diagnoses.

An example of the epistemic fallacy: the false case of "burn-out"

Let us take the true-life example of a middle-aged woman who started to experience general feelings of malaise. These symptoms began to interfere with her capacity to work. She went to a general practitioner and was diagnosed as having "burn-out", that is, it was assumed that her illness was due to stress, and indeed, her symptoms did "tick the boxes" for this diagnosis. The doctor prescribed rest and a job change. However, her symptoms did not abate, but became worse. She became incapable of eating, dressing, washing herself, etc. During this two-year-long deterioration, she regularly attended consultations with her doctor, but the original diagnosis was never questioned. However, she occasionally expressed a deep dissatisfaction with her treatment and uncertainty of the diagnosis. After two years, her family decided to act because they suspected that the diagnosis was wrong. They took the initiative because the woman had become incapable of acting on her own behalf. They demanded a reappraisal of her case, asking that it be carried out without any preconceptions. The resulting appraisal admitted that her symptoms "indicated an Alzheimer-like symptomology", but a diagnosis was withheld (i.e. the health establishment refused to commit themselves to agreeing that her Alzheimer's disease actually, ontologically, existed). Sadly, the woman continued to deteriorate and later passed away.

This story shows how the epistemic fallacy, which results in the hypostatization of symptoms (seeing them as the actual disease), can blind practitioners to the truth of a health problem, resulting in inappropriate or delayed interventions. In this case, despite evidence that their diagnosis was wrong, the health practitioners representing the health establishment did not look more broadly for other evidence that might help them to provide a better diagnosis, neither did they adequately compare the competing theories of the underlying causal mechanisms (they did not use judgemental rationality and the process of elimination). They did not make use of the evidence that their interventions were not working, suggesting an incorrect diagnosis, because there was no box to tick for this. This particular box (whether interventions have worked) is frequently left out due to the over-confidence that comes from assuming that the measurements of the disease are the disease (hypostasis), which is a consequence of the epistemic fallacy.

DSM-5 and its fictive placeholders

The problem of the reification of symptoms is often discussed in relation to the Diagnostic and Statistical Manual of Mental Disorders (DSM) currently in its fifth edition (American Psychiatric Association, 2013). Earlier versions of the DSM clearly warned against reification. For instance, the DSM–4 (American Psychiatric Association, 1994) acknowledged that, "There is no assumption that each category of mental disorder is a completely discrete entity with absolute boundaries dividing it from other mental disorders or from no mental disorder" (xxxi). However, according to Nussbaum (2013) the disclaimer that the categorization of the disorders should not be taken as absolute was disingenuous and similar to the way that a shop proprietor sells rolling papers to an adolescent customer with a knowing wink, reminding him that "this product is not to be used with any illegal substances". We would say that this problem, of mentioning reification but nevertheless proceeding to reify, is typical when no alternative is provided. Critical realism provides just such an alternative with its idea that categories are transfactuals and that although concrete universal categories exist, these are expressed at the level of the empirical as concrete singulars, which are always significantly and uniquely mediated by open-system factors (cf. Chapter 7).

Unlike earlier DSM editions, which were ambiguous about reification, the DSM-5 attempts to avoid reification by stating that its categories are "fictive placeholders", awaiting validation from biological markers (Nussbaum, 2013). As we explained in Chapter 7, no one can be taken seriously if they truly think that what they say is fictional. It is therefore not surprising that the DSM-5 is not taken seriously by some; for instance, the National Institute of Mental Health has refused to use the DSM-5 categories for research purposes (Nussbaum, 2013). What has happened is that in the absence of the acknowledgement that reality is layered and emergent, the authors of the DSM-5 have had to assume that their ideas of transfactual categories – which refer to an emergent, non-empirical reality, specifically emergent from the behaviours of actual patients – have no ontology and are consequently fictional. Therefore, their only justification for using categories is to say that they serve a utilitarian purpose (one cannot justify them by showing that they are real). The DSM-5 is therefore an excellent example of the pomo flips described by Sayer (2000) in which a commentator flips between the extremes of empiricism (the DSM-5 is committed to reducing psychological dysfunctions to empirical, biological "tick box" markers) and postmodernist relativism (the DSM-5 admits that in the absence of such biological markers, it is forced to use categories that are fictions and merely have a utilitarian function). Unfortunately, in practice, this results in entrenching the "tick-box" approach to symptoms and diagnoses, with all of its attendant risks.

The third enigma: What causes it?

A problem with the mainstream approach to causation (what causes it) is that positivist scientists have two philosophies: a diurnal one, namely the philosophy implicit in their spontaneous practice; and a nocturnal one, namely the philosophy that they espouse when they self-consciously reflect on their practice (Bhaskar 2009: 224). From a critical realist perspective, this makes our critique of scientists' praxis difficult because it must be carefully qualified. We can say that "scientists do not value transfactual theories of causation", but the scientists will be quick to point out that they *do* use transfactual theory in their practice. So perhaps instead we need to say that in their nocturnal philosophy, they do not value transfactual explanations and the rational process of elimination that allows scientists to prefer a particular theory over other competing theories. However, in their diurnal philosophy, transfactual theories and the process of elimination are often very important. The reason that the nocturnal philosophy sometimes translates into the absence of transfactual theory in the diurnal philosophy is that, since the presence of transfactual theorizing as part of scientific method is not formal, it becomes optional, and therefore provides strategic advantages to those with ideological agendas. For instance, if a transfactual theory suggests an inconvenient truth, the researchers can simply ignore it (cf. Chapter 14). If an inconvenient truth does get published, opponents can accuse it of being unscientific and unproven (as we have seen in the climate change debate).

This third enigma is associated with the explanatory logic of retroduction (R). Traditionally, this question has been addressed through correlations. However, in contrast to mainstream science, critical realism insists that it is not enough to know that A is correlated to B to assume that A causes B; it is also necessary to develop a transfactual theory of the structures and mechanisms (at the level of the real) that cause the problem and to eliminate (E) competing transfactual theories. Transfactual causation in the open system of our world is enigmatic because it is fallible: there is always a chance that further evidence will require us to adjust our theories. Once one breaks from the need to justify knowledge purely in terms of the empirical or the actual – that is, once one considers reality to be layered and agrees that we can use interdisciplinary transfactuality to know about the real structures and mechanisms – it is then possible to engage with any significant chunk of reality, no matter how complex. Typically, from a monodisciplinary perspective, when we ask the question "What causes it?" we are looking for a biophysical cause. However, from an interdisciplinary perspective, "What causes it?" is a much bigger question.

An interdisciplinary explanation of diabetes

We can think about this in terms of diabetes. Diabetes is not just a physical disease – it is also a lifestyle issue, having to do with the economic structure of society and exposure to adverts and other information that leads to detrimental eating and lifestyle. Diabetes is a good example of the way in which social context is important in causal genesis. In general, if there is not a biomedical basis for a condition, the medical professions tend to side-line it; perhaps their reason for this is the view (or feeling) – which may be wrong – that they can do nothing or very little about it. A useful heuristic to guide interdisciplinary research that aims to go beyond the reduction of causation to the biophysical is the seven laminations of scale (cf. Chapter 5). At each lamination there are different mechanisms, playing different roles (e.g. some predisposing and some triggering). The exact weight of the different mechanisms and how the levels mesh together may vary from case to case, so that there is not only a conjunctive multiplicity, but also a disjunctive plurality, of causes – in other words you not only have A and B and C, but also X or Y or Z. In a critical realist summary and analysis of the literature, Daniel Seldén (2005) argues for an interdisciplinary pluralistic methodological approach informed by a stratified pluralistic ontology, in which the specific methodology will be different for each level. Table 10.1 gives an incomplete (merely illustrative) interdisciplinary explanation for the preconditions and causal structures and mechanisms of diabetes based on Bhaskar's seven laminations of scale.

Despite this consensus on the need for a multi-perspectival approach, attempts to develop it usually flounder. In short, the need for an integral approach is acknowledged in theory but this rarely translates into practice. For the most part, researchers from different disciplines tend to remain narrowly focused on the mechanisms in their disciplines. For instance, if we consider anorexia nervosa, in neuropsychiatry, the focus is on neuropeptides and monoamine systems. In social anthropology, the focus is on the notion of body ideals prevalent in the culture of the West. In social science, the focus is on risk factors, or correlations, of which three have been identified as important: psychopathological disturbances or disorders in the family; the social position of the family (for instance divorced parents or very young parents); and the family dynamics or interactions. Furthermore, it seems that there are: factors which predispose; factors which trigger or release (induce); and factors (mechanisms) which sustain. Some researchers claim that there is a genetic predisposition to anorexia, while others say there is an interplay of mechanisms that bring on the emergence of anorexia and that genetic predispositions are not strictly necessary. Even if the genetic predisposition is fairly strong, the intent or will of the person who has anorexia is still part of the causation. The lesson here (and one which we will discuss more later) is that when we translate our understanding of causes into action for prevention or healing, success is less likely if we have a reductionist view of the situation.

"What causes it?" becomes the thing itself

Another important point is that there is a strong connection between the question "What is it?" and the question "What causes it?" because typically our knowledge of a subject progresses in such a way that the explanation for something becomes the thing itself, that is, it becomes the "something" that needs further explanation. This happens at the Identification (I) stage of the DREI(C). We have already described how the explanation for water, that it is made of hydrogen and oxygen, has become a way to identify or describe water (as H_2O) (cf. Chapter 6). This is also true of health issues. If we take the issue of the dramatic increase in mortality rates in the UK in 2015 (Donnelly, 2016), the question "What is it?" – answer: high mortality rates – has quickly become a question of "What causes it?" – answer: a bad strain of

TABLE 10.1 An interdisciplinary explanation for the causal mechanisms of diabetes

Bhaskar's seven laminations of scale	Causal mechanisms of type 2 diabetes
(i) the sub-individual level	E.g. at the biophysical level, a lack of insulin in the body causes diabetes. However, other sub-individual mechanisms may also be relevant; for instance major depressive disorders may have a role and seem to increase the risk for onset of type II diabetes (Polonsky et al., 2005). Also, some people have a genetic predisposition to diabetes (Horenstein and Shuldiner, 2004).
(ii) the individual or biographical level	E.g. an inverse relationship exists between social position and incidence of diabetes (Kumari, Head and Marmot, 2004).
(iii) the micro-level studied, for example, by ethnomethodologists and others	E.g. research has shown that potentially modifiable risk factors in African Americans, related to lifestyle issues common to this group, lead to a substantially increased risk of diabetes (Brancati et al., 2000).
(iv) the meso-level at which we are concerned with the relations between functional roles	E.g. the micro-level lifestyle characteristics of African Americans, that increase the risk of diabetes, are partly explainable in terms of structural relations of racism (Karlsen and Nazroo, 2002). The experience of racism is related to increased risk of diabetes in African Americans (Moody-Ayers et al., 2005).
(v) the macro-level orientated to the understanding of the functioning of whole societies or their regions	E.g. Aschner et al. (2014) relate certain characteristics of the populations of South and Central America to the issue of diabetes (such as rates of obesity).
(vi) the mega-level of the analysis of whole traditions and civilizations	E.g. the UK has a well-established tradition of entrenched classism that has consequences for a variety of health issues, including the increased incidence of diabetes in deprived classes (Connolly et al., 2000).
(vii) the planetary (or cosmological) level concerned with the planet (or cosmos) as a whole	E.g. a consequence of globalization is a worldwide increase in Western diets and sedentary habits, which have been associated with a rise in diabetes. This has been well-documented in China (Hu, 2011).

flu, an ineffective flu vaccination and a rise in the elderly population, and/or perhaps reduced health and social services (Mundasad, 2016; Garthwaite, 2014).

The fourth enigma: What cures (or at least alleviates) it?

Bhaskar (2008b/1993: 261–262) makes the point that once we have explained a problem, then, *ceteris paribus* (all other things being equal), we can move directly to a relevant action, based on a negative evaluation of the cause and a positive evaluation of any action designed to absent it. However, this is not always a simple matter. For example, we have a rather good understanding of the processes behind HIV/AIDS but at the moment we have no effective way of curing it. The obvious action, based on a negative evaluation of the presence of HIV, is to remove the HIV from the infected person, but this is easier to say than to do. It can also be the other way around. For example, we have not found the deeper causes of rheumatoid arthritis (Hensvold et al., 2013) but we have been able to develop drugs that are highly effective in alleviating its symptoms.

Curing and alleviating as retrodictive back-casting

When we are looking for ways to cure or alleviate a disease, and we already know what causes it, then we are engaging in applied science (cf. Chapter 5). Invention and creativity often play an important part here, since we will need to invent a solution to cure something or to ameliorate its effects. To do this, scientists use the logic of retrodiction in a certain way. Typically, retrodiction is the use of established theory to explain how things *must have been* for things to be as they are now. However, to find a cure, scientists use established theory to explain how things *might be* in order to achieve some imagined future good. Retrodiction in this conception is still a logic of the past (hence it is still "retro") but now the scientists imagine themselves at some future point where the disease is healed and ask what must have happened to have resulted in the healing, using established theory to answer their question. This process has also been called back-casting (Holmberg and Robèrt, 2000). For example, once we knew what caused diabetes (the absence of insulin) we were able to use retrodictive back-casting to arrive at the idea of introducing insulin into the blood of diabetic patients to alleviate their condition. This brought its own set of creative challenges, and required interdisciplinary collaboration. For instance, there was the need for: bio-engineering, to make the insulin; product design engineering, to make the containers to transport the insulin and the instruments to administer it; and social science interventions, to address the factors that might impede patient adherence to their medical regime.

Explaining clinical trial results and side-effects using retrodiction

In the process of arriving at a biophysical cure or treatment, scientists are likely to use clinical trials. Again, applied science and its associated logic of retrodiction are important here. For example, in clinical trials involving the administration of different quantities of insulin, the scientists would have retrodictively used their theory of how the insulin is used by the body to explain their results. If certain phenomena occurred as side-effects, such as hypoglycaemic events, the scientists would have been able to retrodictively explain these in terms of their theory. In this case, the theory of the role played by insulin in blood glucose levels tells us that glucose levels can fall after administering insulin, in the absence of a meal, as the insulin then removes too much glucose from the blood.

Finally, applied research to find a cure or to alleviate a disease results in *Identification* of all the relevant components of the problem. In this process, we increase our confidence that the issue really exists since our theory of it should explain relatively small features of it. We also evaluate the outcomes of our applied interventions, to check the theory. If our research at the *Identification* stage results in anomalies not explained by the original theory – such as pieces of the situation that the theory cannot explain or unexpected outcomes of interventions – this requires that we correct it, which is the *Correction* phase of the RRREI(C).

The fifth enigma: What prevents it?

This enigma has been poorly understood because of the way that mainstream irrealist science denies ontological status to the non-empirical. It therefore relies on shallow empirical correlations to provide predictions about the future. This can lead to:

1. *Misjudgements and policy mistakes* (e.g. a discussion follows of how health advisors may have mistakenly recommended the reduction of dietary saturated fat and cholesterol-reducing statins to prevent heart disease).
2. *Instrumental approaches to prevention*, with little hope of dealing with the deeper causes of the issues (e.g. a discussion then follows of the use of "risk factors" to devise policy to prevent gender-based violence).
3. *Preventative inaction* in the face of evidence that gives an imperative to act preventatively (e.g. a discussion follows last of the way that mainstream scientific method has led to our failure to act to prevent climate change despite excellent evidence that indicates the urgency of such action).

Preventing heart disease

It is tempting for policy-makers to rely on correlations to justify preventative interventions because, despite the well-acknowledged critique of this approach, there is no alternative to it in mainstream science. For example, it is standard medical practice to assume that the intake of saturated fat and low density lipid (LDL) cholesterol must be controlled to reduce the risk of cardiovascular disease. However, in the *British Medical Journal (BMJ)*, Malhotra (2013) explains that this advice may have paradoxically increased cardiovascular risk because it has increased the intake of sugar which can cause metabolic syndrome. He also claims that "the government's obsession with levels of total cholesterol" has led to the overmedication of millions of people with statins. He explains further:

> Saturated fat has been demonised ever since Ancel Keys's landmark "seven countries" study in 1970. This concluded that a correlation existed between

the incidence of coronary heart disease and total cholesterol concentrations, which then correlated with the proportion of energy provided by saturated fat. But correlation is not causation.

(Malhotra, 2013: 347)

This problem was made possible because of the medical establishment's over-reliance on correlation statistics, resulting in their reification of cholesterol as a risk factor in heart disease. There is a good chance that this would not have happened if there had been a scientific norm, such as we advocate here, that insisted: (a) such correlations are only taken as causal once we can explain them using transfactual theory based on a broad spread of evidence from different sources; and (b) such a transfactual theory is only taken seriously after it has been subjected to an extensive comparison against competing theories. This is because, when a scientist begins to look for a transfactual explanation for an observation or correlation, it is likely that there will be information missing or absent. These absences need to be absented, to provide a full-enough description of the situation. Additionally, a transfactual theory is judged to be better than its competitors in terms of how much of the broad evidence it manages to explain. This means that it must embrace all of what is already known and should not limit itself to correlation knowledge. In the case of the advice that we should reduce dietary saturated fat, there was information that contradicted this advice, such as "the French paradox". This is the paradox that the French, who have low coronary heart disease death rates, nevertheless have a high intake of dietary cholesterol and saturated fat (Ferrières, 2004). In Humean empiricist scientific methodology, descriptive statistics are the poor cousin of correlational statistics, as correlations are assumed to be the best way to determine causation. However, in critical realist science, descriptive statistics (such as epidemiological studies) and even one-off events are valued along with correlational statistics because of their ability to support or disconfirm transfactual theories of causation (see also Chapter 14). In the process of the establishment of a law of nature based on a correlation, three questions must be asked (Bhaskar, 2008a/1975: 164):

i   Does such a correlation exist, that might constitute the basis for a law? (Description)
ii Is there some reason, other than the correlation, for why the factors involved in the correlation should be related? (Retroduction and Elimination)
iii Is this reason located in the enduring powers of things and the transfactually active mechanisms of nature? (Identification)

If the answer to (i) is yes we have what might be called a "protolaw". Typically, mainstream empiricist scientists are content to prematurely terminate their scientific endeavour after achieving a shallow protolaw; in the case of cholesterol, they were content that there was a strong correlation between cholesterol levels and cardiovascular disease. There was no formal requirement for scientists to provide a transfactual theory explaining the correlation, although they did in fact supply such a theory in the form of the idea that the cholesterol formed plaques on the side of arteries, leading to arteriosclerosis. Because there was no formal requirement for this transfactual theory to be compared to competing theories (the DREI(C)'s Elimination phase), this theory remained unquestioned and served as a psychological prop to justify the policy interventions derived from the correlation. In fact, there *was* at least one other competing transfactual theory, namely that the cholesterol was present in high concentrations at the sites of arteriosclerosis because it formed a protective wall around damaged areas of arteries. For example, Kaunitz (1977, 1978) suggested that the strong correlation between arteriosclerosis and high-serum cholesterol might not be causal. Instead, the cholesterol-based atheroma tissue may have a healing function, since the composition of the atheroma is the same as for many granulation tissues which, in other contexts, are associated with healing processes. He stated:

> Such a hypothesis could explain all the well-known arteriosclerotic changes. Long term studies in man for testing the serum cholesterol-lowering action of the "unsaturated" vegetable oils include serious errors of method and permit no confirmed conclusions.
>
> (Kaunitz, 1977: 539)

Kaunitz's accusations of "serious errors of method" were largely ignored because the errors to which he referred were based on mainstream science's culturally entrenched reification of correlations. Another reason that mainstream scientists failed to admit that there were potential problems with their theory was because there was no formal requirement for them to use the results of any interventions as further evidence to feed back into their scientific enterprise (the Correction phase of the DREIC). In the instance of the use of statins to prevent heart disease, the UK's National Institute for Health and Care Excellence (NICE) recommends that statin therapy is provided as primary prevention for those individuals without known cardiovascular disease but who have an estimated 10-year risk of developing cardiovascular disease of at least 10% (Collins et al., 2016). However, Malhotra (2013) explains that despite 60 million statin prescriptions a year in the UK, it is difficult to demonstrate at the population level any additional effect of statins on reduced cardiovascular mortality over the effects of the decline in smoking prevalence and primary angioplasty. A rebuttal of this claim – that there is questionable significant benefit in the widespread use of statins for primary prevention, that is, for people who show no signs of cardiovascular disease – has been supplied by Collins et al. (2016) but their argument is unconvincing if one looks at it carefully. For instance, they concede that typical statin use for primary prevention will provide only a 0.3–0.6% reduction in possible heart events per year (1.5–3%, or 150–300 events per 10,000, per 5 years); and that this slight advantage is to some extent offset by a 0.2–0.4% increase in adverse effects per year, including new-onset diabetes, which ironically is itself associated with an increase in heart disease (there is less controversy around the benefits of statins for secondary prevention, which is associated with significantly higher reduction in heart disease). Collins et al. (2016) also concede that statins raise blood glucose levels and increase concentrations of liver enzymes. Furthermore, they admit that in older people there is a negative association between cholesterol and mortality (lower cholesterol levels are associated with greater mortality, though they say that this is not causal), and that healthy people tend to have higher levels of cholesterol (pre-existing disease is associated with low levels of cholesterol). These last two correlations are anomalies, like the French paradox, that need to be incorporated into a broad, interdisciplinary explanation of the role of cholesterol in health and wellbeing. Problematically, Collins et al. do not attempt to explain the empirical evidence using a transfactual theory. They base their argument on correlations alone. That is, they do not take the further step in their analysis from a protolaw to a retroductive theory about the deeper causes and mechanisms of the role of cholesterol (and therefore cholesterol-lowering statins) on human health and wellbeing. It is also perhaps relevant that cholesterol is necessary for vitamin D production; and it has been demonstrated that there is a positive correlation between the amount of vitamin D made by the body during sun exposure and available levels of cholesterol (Bogh et al., 2010). Perhaps cholesterol initially plays a positive role, but only becomes problematic (blocking arteries) when vascular problems become excessive (which would explain why statins are clearly helpful for secondary prevention of heart disease but are not so clearly helpful for primary prevention). Although it is not our objective to provide an alternative transfactual theory for the role of cholesterol in heart disease, we suggest that there is perhaps a trade-off between the advantages and disadvantages of relatively high cholesterol.

Encouragingly, at the time of writing, there is a debate in progress, led by the medical journals *The Lancet* and the *BMJ*, on the value of the last 50 years of medical recommendations based on the assumption that lower cholesterol reduces heart disease. This advice has been used to justify the widespread prescription of statins as a preventative measure. While one *Lancet* article, written by researchers closely associated with pharmaceutical companies, makes the case for the continued preventative use of statins (Collins et al., 2016), another article in the *BMJ* has called for an independent investigation into the problem (Godlee, 2016). The stakes are high; statins are widely known to be hugely profitable for pharmaceutical companies. In 2016, they were the most prescribed medication in the world (Hobbs et al., 2016). Significantly, both proponents and opponents of the extensive use of statins have avoided transfactual retroductive theories to support their position, remaining faithful to the Humean empiricist paradigm in which correlations are questionably assumed to be both necessary and sufficient to justify assumptions of causation. This controversy would benefit from a critical realist approach to science.

Preventing gender-based violence

An example of how interdisciplinary components of prevention are reduced to empirical risk factors is provided by the World Health Organization's (2010) interdisciplinary advice on the prevention of gender-based violence. The risk factors include: low income; low education; sexual abuse as a child; intra-parental violence; anti-social personality disorders; harmful use of alcohol and drugs; acceptance of violence; multiple partners/infidelity; low resistance to peer pressure; weak community sanctions; poverty; traditional gender norms; and social norms supportive of violence. Note that these factors are not used as evidence to support interacting transfactual theories of the causal mechanisms of gender-based violence. Instead, they are used to justify instrumental preventative measures that include behaviour-changing education campaigns against, for instance, alcohol abuse and the social acceptance of violence. However, simply providing behaviour-change messages, without dealing with the underlying reasons, motives, and opportunities for the unwanted behaviour, is notoriously unlikely to be effective (Ryan and Deci, 2008).

If we instead attempt to take a multimechanism approach to the issue of gender-based violence, considering specifically South Africa, where rates of gender-based violence are some of the highest in the world, there are a number of possible transfactual theories of mechanisms that may be relevant. This results in a more nuanced approach to preventative measures. For instance, we might consider, among other things, four possible mechanisms that explain the correlations and other evidence (here we are not attempting to be comprehensive but merely illustrative; neither are we necessarily advocating these interventions).

Mechanism 1: For instance, poverty is a risk factor, but is this because of the mechanism by which women have no economic alternatives to remaining with abusers? If so, then providing safe-houses and financial support to women to give them a chance to get on their own feet may be more effective than an overall decrease in poverty, especially if the latter is achieved by increasing wealth controlled by men.

Mechanism 2: Furthermore, is the poverty merely an exacerbating consequence of a deeper problem of capitalist labour markets that isolate individuals, removing them from their support networks, resulting in a mechanism for violence which is that individuals are not encouraged by other community members to either refrain from, or refuse to accept, violence? If poverty is an exacerbating consequence of current labour policies, and we try to remove it by more vigorously applying those same labour policies, we run the risk of making the problem worse.

Mechanism 3: There is a correlation between alcoholism and violence against women. Is the alcohol causal, or is it too an exacerbating consequence of social imbalances? Are men drinking to cope with the stress of their lives? Instrumentally increasing taxes on alcohol and providing media messages against drinking may not help if the underlying motivation to drink, the mechanism for it, is not addressed; for instance, men may simply turn instead to illegal alcohol. This may make the situation worse since illegal alcohol is unregulated and therefore potentially more intoxicating. Alternatively, men may not stop drinking, but because of the taxes may have to put more of their wages towards the purchase of alcohol, resulting in an overall increase in poverty, again exacerbating the problem.

Mechanism 4: Currently, men are simplistically considered mainly to blame for the violence and thus become the focus of the intervention – we want them to change their behaviour without asking why they are behaving in these ways in the first place. However, a theory exists that suggests that a causal mechanism of the abuse is that South African black men, as well as women, are experiencing oppression and that the men who perpetrate violence are themselves trying to cope with both historical and current racism (Price, 2010). If this is the case, then perhaps we need to support men as well as women to prevent abuse.

This is not to say that instrumental preventative measures are not sometimes useful in the short term, but that the absence of a multimechanism analysis risks interventions that lead to unintended consequences and fail to address the underlying causes. Notice too, how the four mechanisms suggested address issues at the seven levels of scale (cf. Chapter 5), ranging from the global to the psychological levels. In other words, scientists need to move away from basing preventative measures on protolaws and instead base their preventative measures on retroductively derived interdisciplinary theories of mechanisms and structures.

Preventative inaction: the case of our failure to prevent climate change

Most scientists are happy to accept the evidence at hand that climate change – which potentially risks the wellbeing of all – is both anthropogenic and serious enough to warrant immediate and far-reaching preventative action (Oreskes, 2007). However, as already mentioned in Chapter 7 (Step 3), most conservative politicians in the UK and the USA agree that it has not yet been conclusively proved that climate change is manmade. They agree with Bratby (2010), that climate change science is a poor basis for action because it is not based on falsifiable hypotheses. However, as far as critical realists are concerned, it is possible to develop scientific knowledge in contexts where one cannot carry out falsifiable, closed-system experiments. In such contexts, we use *Retroduction* to identify antecedent causes and we validate our findings through the process of judgemental rationality and *Elimination*. This means that the critical realist position may be able to justify taking action sooner than is currently the norm because it allows us to take seriously our theories about causal mechanisms even if these are not able to be experimentally or empirically verified. If one is an empiricist, and thus assumes (because one does not have the methodological tools to insist otherwise) that the causal theory in question is an untested correlation describing simplistic cause and effect, then taking such a liberty seems irresponsible, and indeed it is. However, if the theory in question is a transfactual one, based on extensive and interdisciplinary evidence (such as the theory of climate change), then it would be irresponsible not to act on it.

The sixth enigma: How is it experienced?

We need to answer the question "How is it experienced?" from both an ontological and an epistemological perspective. Ontologically speaking, the question refers us to the realm of the concrete singular, since every individual's experience is a unique instantiation of concrete universal structures as a result of differentiating mediations and rhythmics (Bhaskar, 2008b/1993: 132). This means that for any particular illness, the way that it is experienced will depend on such differentiating factors as the person's age, ethnicity, life history, genetic make-up, psychological disposition, access to resources, and social standing. Furthermore, the experience of the illness will differ over time, perhaps as the result of the typical progression of the disease, or simply as the person ages. Recognition of the way that every person is unique has resulted in the move within the medical profession towards individualizing treatments, sometimes known as Mutually Agreed Tailoring (Denford et al., 2014). Of course, the concrete universal can also change over time, so for example, the concrete universal that is the disease of HIV has changed over time due to differentiating mediations that include the way that the virus has mutated, advances in treatment and prevention, and changes in the public perception of the disease. This results in the need to consider any concrete universal as a multiple quadruplicity, consisting of changing: (1) structures; (2) mediations; (3) singularities; and (4) processes.

From an epistemological or transitive perspective, any medical or wellbeing practitioner will usually start by asking the patient about the way that they are experiencing their problem. While this is not always possible, for example, in the case of young children, it is nevertheless an advantage that the medical profession has over many other professions. It is also important to acknowledge that no human being can experience what another human being is experiencing, and therefore – assuming the absence of deceit, to which we will return later – it is safe to say that the patient is the best authority on what they are experiencing. Even when a person is suffering from hallucinations and can see pink elephants – but there are no pink elephants – nevertheless their *belief* that pink elephants are present is real because ontology is maximally inclusive and therefore includes false beliefs (cf. Step 1, Chapter 7).

Our conceptualizations are corrigible but important

However, being able to understand what we are experiencing – our conceptualizations about it – is another matter and critical realism teaches us that, contrary to the hermeneuticist position, people's interpretations or conceptualizations of their situations are corrigible. People may simply be unaware of what is happening to them (lack the advanced concepts required to interpret their symptoms) or they may be afraid to admit to themselves the true situation and thus be experiencing denial (Freudian rationalization). It must also be acknowledged that some patients may purposely deceive medical practitioners, for a number of reasons ranging from a personality disorder to socio-economic fears – such as a loss of wages if they go to hospital. Because of this potential for corrigibility, it is important that diagnosis is based on both the patients' verbalized experience and corroborating evidence. Nevertheless, "the low status given to experience in the hierarchy of evidence" has been identified as an important limiting factor in providing person-centred health care (Greenhalgh et al., 2015). Note that lacking advanced concepts to interpret a set of symptoms, or Freudian rationalization, is not limited to the patients; they can be associated with the medical practitioner too. Therefore, reflexivity and an attitude of lifelong learning are a necessary part of one's professional practice (cf. Step 5, Chapter 7).

The seventh enigma: How are we to alleviate and cure it?

This enigma expresses the healing function of medicine and has to do with intervention, treatment, therapy, and rehabilitation. In this book we think that it is ethically and logically preferable to see the patient as the agent of their own healing, although this does not deny the agency of the medical practitioner; it merely places the practitioner into a supportive role. Conceptually, it is important to appreciate from the outset that any ill related to wellbeing can be considered to be an absence, and any absence can be seen as a constraint. Thus we have the metatheorem: ills → absences → constraints. Inasmuch as these constraints are (i) unwanted, (ii) unnecessary, and (iii) remediable or removable, the objective should be to transformatively negate them, i.e. absent them. The opposite of a constraint is both "freedom from" and "freedom to" and the root conception of freedom is that of "autonomy" in the sense of self-determination. Rational autonomy includes cognitive, empowered, and dispositional or motivational aspects (Bhaskar, 2008b/1993: 260). Therefore, in order for a person to possess rational agency they must:

i   possess the knowledge to act in their own real interests (the cognitive requirement);
ii be able to access the skill, resources, and opportunities to do so (the empowered component); and
iii be disposed to so act (the dispositional or motivational condition).

Of course the "knowledge" mentioned in (i) may be practical, tacit knowledge rather than theoretical knowledge (knowledge "how" rather than knowledge "that"). Cognitively, it is possible that a person may lack the desire to be free from an ill because they do not know that they suffer from it (for instance, a first step in healing from alcoholism is to acknowledge that one suffers from the disease). Conversely, a person may desire to be free from an ill, but lack the concrete power and/or knowledge to achieve this, for example, perhaps they lack access to health care or literacy. Furthermore, they may satisfy criteria (i) and (ii), that is, they may have the knowledge and the resources to act, but they may lack the disposition to act (perhaps they are severely depressed or feel discouraged).

Healing as praxis: a case study of anorexia

In Step 4, Chapter 7, Bhaskar suggests a format for the emancipatory dialectic as transformed, transformative, totalizing, transformist (TTTT$_\varnothing$) praxis. We illustrate this now with a fictional female character with anorexia whose path to healing therefore involves, iteratively:

i   Transformed (autoplastic [cf. 1M non-identity]) – absences in one's self are absented; and
ii   Transformative (alloplastic [cf. 2E negativity]) – one has the resources to embark on a dialectic of change to one's environment and surroundings, including in terms of one's relationships with other people (absenting absences).

Since there is a coincidence of autoplastic and alloplastic change (changes in oneself coincide with changes in the world), we will deal with points (i) and (ii) together. To begin with, as a first step to healing, a woman suffering from anorexia nervosa might acknowledge that she has a serious condition (autoplastic – absences the absence of her acknowledgement of a problem). She then goes to the doctor to get resources to help herself (alloplastic – absences the absence of help and resources). As a result, she begins taking potassium supplements and hormones to increase her oestrogen levels (autoplastic – absences the absence of potassium and oestrogen in her body). However, there may be limits to the objective potential for healing, i.e. there is always a possible disjuncture between subjective needs and objective potential. For instance, she may want to get psychological counselling, but her insurance may not cover mental health.

iii Totalizing (all-inclusive and auto-reflexive [cf. 3L totality or reflexivity]) – one is able to immerse oneself in the totality and reflexively consider what it is about the situation that constrains achieving wholeness.

The anorexic woman discovers that the initial element of her illness is reflected, in different ways, into other elements of the totality of her life and emergent society (significantly in this case, patriarchal society that objectifies women's bodies in a certain way). She therefore begins to think of the totality of her existence as an intra-actively changing embedded ensemble (her inter-active, changing roles as a daughter and employee, embedded in wider patriarchal society), constituted by her geohistory and/or its traces (she is a second-generation American whose Irish family emigrated to the USA) and her context (her family are strict religious fundamentalists). Hepworth (1999) outlines the different social, cultural, and feminist theories of anorexia nervosa, explaining how they have changed over time and reflecting the consensus that we need an interdisciplinary approach to dealing with anorexia. She stresses the connection between the mother–daughter relationship, patriarchal social structure, and the denial of nutrition needs; and she sees anorexia as an attempt to exert control in the construction of the person's own identity (see Table 10.2).

The way that the individual (concrete singular) is embedded in the totality explains why anorexia affects some individuals and not others, and why it affects

The seven enigmas of healing 109

TABLE 10.2 Examples of mechanisms relevant to anorexia at different levels of reality

Level	Mechanisms (examples)
Socio-cultural	Ethnicity, class, sex, relations in the family, social identity, slim ideal, discourses
Psychological	Cognition, learning, dysfunctional pattern of mind, childhood trauma, incautious fantasies, inner conflicts, symbolic actions
Biological	Biological constraints, the anatomy of the brain, transmitter substances, genetic factors

Source: adapted from Seldén (2005: 64).

them differently. At the level of the concrete singular, the concrete universal conjunctive multiplicity of mechanisms will play out with differing degrees of weight (for example, the important role of media images will play out differently in different individuals depending on their access to the images or the images' place in their particular culture) and some mechanisms may not be relevant at all due to open-system factors (for example, episodes of bulimia may not be possible if someone lives at home, due to parental surveillance, but this may change when they go to college). The disjunctive plurality necessary to provide a concrete universal theory of anorexia (such as the acknowledgement that it is common among both straight women and gay men) will be distilled down to only one of the mutually exclusive possibilities in the concrete singular (i.e. one is either a straight woman or a gay man).

The agent's totalizing process – their path towards understanding how they are embedded in the totality – will be open-ended and potentially disjointed. It results in reflexivity and perspective switches, in which the narrative of the anorexic's life must be continually rewritten and social landscapes remapped. For instance, the woman with anorexia kept a journal and described how at first she did not have a name for her illness. She described her writing as "the confused ravings of a tired, sad, angry person". When she was given her diagnosis – and her illness now had a name – it "changed things". Suddenly her symptoms were not puzzling or unique but corresponded to a wider cultural narrative that anorexia was about needing to be in control and about rebellion against parents/society/femininity/patriarchy. She incorporated these descriptions and explanations into her own narrative, at first not knowing that it was possible to create something different. Her healing began in earnest when she began to tell a different narrative, one of her transition towards health.

iv Transformist – one's action is oriented to structural change, informed by the explanatory critique developed in (iii) and concrete utopianism (cf. 4D agency).

As the anorexic woman began to grow in her self-esteem, she began to refuse structural sexism in her home or at work (where this was possible). If she was unable to renegotiate her life politics with certain individuals in order to achieve mutual self-esteem, she distanced herself from them. She joined a feminist group and made a point of reminding her female friends of the importance of voting. Eventually she broadened her focus from feminist concerns to a more general emancipatory politics, oriented towards universal human flourishing (for an outline of the relationship between the concrete singular and political activity see Figure 10.1). This later stage is important because "the development of the concrete singularity of each, is a condition of the concrete singularity of all" (paraphrasing Marx, in Bhaskar, 2008b/1993: 372), which is also why the title of this book contains the term *wellbeing* instead of *health*; the latter provides an overly narrow, monodisciplinary view of human flourishing. In a eudaimonic situation, all will be free from constraints, that is, all will be both free from ills and free to pursue their life goals.

The opposite of this interdisciplinary path to healing (agency) is: the continued presence of absence → alterity (disconnectedness) → de-totalization (alienating split-off or marginalization) → impotent self. Bhaskar (2008b/1993) later added two more Ts to the TTTT$_\varnothing$ to make it TTTTTT. After the final T, and instead of the $_\varnothing$, he added *Transitional*. After the *Totalizing*, he added *Trustworthy*. The latter addition is necessary because it is possible for the narratives that we tell ourselves and others to be deceitful. For example, perhaps we tell ourselves and our doctor that we need a gastric band. But, is this really true? And is it worth the risk of surgery? (It is important to consider issues of existential security.) If it is not true, have we considered the waste of National Health Service resources, or the waste of the surgeon's time? (It is important to consider ergonic efficiency.) Perhaps it would be better to empower ourselves by emancipating ourselves from those behaviours that lead to our weight problems. (It is important to be empowered.)

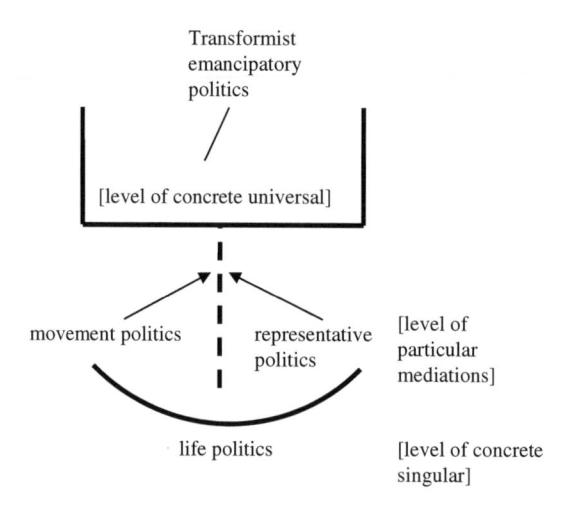

FIGURE 10.1 Transformist politics
Source: Bhaskar (2008b/1993: 267).

Furthermore, we cannot consider our actions apart from their effect on others, in this case, the other people on waiting lists for surgery (universal emancipation). Clearly, sometimes a gastric band is the best solution, but the point here is that we need to be honest with ourselves and others (trustworthy).

As the previous example shows, totalizing praxis requires stretching the moral imagination. However, only the empowered individual can assist or effectively solidarize with the powerless. It is therefore enlightening and not egoistic for the individual to acknowledge her real self-interests. In the gastric band example, if – after reflexively assessing the options and their consequences – we decide that a gastric band is indeed necessary for us to achieve our full potential, this is not necessarily egoistic if it results in our flourishing. This leads Bhaskar (2008b/1993: 120) to provide the objectives of totalizing praxis, which he envisages as a dialectic of 7 E's, all of which have been implied previously:

> self-esteem ↔ mutual esteem (where the intra-dependence of action itself reflects both the fiduciary nature of the social bond and the reality of oppressive social relations) ↔ existential security ↔ ergonic efficiency ↔ (individual → collective → totalizing) empowerment ↔ universal emancipation ↔ eudaimonia.

To conclude, and to place this process of healing into the general dialectic of the MELD (1M, 2E, 3D, 4L, described in Step 2, Chapter 7), we can say that, to achieve healing, it is necessary to *diagnose* the problem, *explain* it, and then take appropriate *action* to absent it. This is the DEA model of practical problem-resolution or reasoning (Bhaskar, 2008b/1993: 261). The DEA model depends on the use of the RRREI(C) model of applied social scientific explanation, which itself depends on iterative applications of the DREI(C) model of pure scientific explanation. In other words, when we diagnose a health problem, we resolve it into its components and then we redescribe it using the appropriate language (for example, we carry out diagnostic tests which allow us to better describe it in terms that allow us to analyse it). We then explain it, by retrodiction, and thus gain an understanding of its antecedent causes. When we use retrodiction (in the process of using the RRREI(C)), we are using already established theories about the multiplicity of relevant mechanisms, which were originally derived from retroduction (in the DREI(C)). It is extremely rare, if ever, that an illness is caused by one mechanism. Usually, it is the result of a large number of interacting mechanisms, such as we have seen in the case of anorexia nervosa. All three models, the DEA (practical problem resolution), and the RRREI(C) and DREI(C) (theoretical problem resolution), are variations of the basic MELD dialectic which is a progression by which an absence or an incompleteness of some sort is rectified (absented). Thus, one moves from an incomplete situation to a more comprehensive totality. As we have already mentioned, the first five enigmas of healing relate to the scientific function of medicine: theoretical problem resolution. Therefore, they are best addressed by the DREI(C) and the RRREI(C). The last two enigmas relate to the second healing function of medicine: practical problem resolution. Therefore, they are best addressed by the DEA.

In the next chapter, we continue with the theme of Part III, which is the practical application of critical realist interdisciplinarity. We will therefore consider the medical profession's use of the concept of the *biopsychosocial*, with special reference to its application in the case of the International Classification of Functioning, Disability and Health (hereafter the ICF). While broadly supportive of the general move towards greater consideration of the biopsychosocial in health and wellbeing contexts, we nevertheless attempt to underlabour for the move by strengthening the argument for it.

11
THE BIOPSYCHOSOCIAL APPROACH, WITH SPECIAL REFERENCE TO THE INTERNATIONAL CLASSIFICATION OF FUNCTIONING, DISABILITY AND HEALTH

Despite the general acceptance of the need for an interdisciplinary approach to health, our clinical practice often fails to reflect this. If anything, it seems that our practice has become increasingly fragmented and specialist over the last three decades. Although a number of case studies show the effectiveness and success of truly interdisciplinary research related to health (e.g. Kessel, Rosenfield and Anderson, 2008), the tendency towards monodisciplinarity remains (e.g. Swedish Research Council (Vetenskapsrådet), 2005; Danermark, 2009). This is not to disparage the great strides that have been made in the specialist spheres, particularly in terms of the development of pharmaceuticals designed to combat particular diseases. However, medical specialization has been sustained by the long-established academic disciplinary divisions and reinforced by funding priorities that prefer discrete research projects over complex interdisciplinary ones, especially if they are empirical, correlative, and laboratory-based.

One of the most common ways to attempt to achieve interdisciplinarity in the medical fields has been through the guidance of the biopsychosocial model, but this has been criticized for several reasons which we will discuss later (Richter, 1999). Nevertheless, despite its limitations, the biopsychosocial model has several redeeming qualities. Therefore, in this chapter, we plan to augment and develop it in a constructive way. In critical realist terms, we will try to underlabour for it, by providing it with a metatheory that can fully support its important aim of interdisciplinarity. Towards the end of the chapter, we will illustrate our argument by applying it to an institution whose principles reflect the main characteristics of the biopsychosocial approach, namely the International Classification of Functioning, Disability and Health (hereafter the ICF).

Introduction to the biopsychosocial model

The biopsychosocial model was first suggested by George Engel in 1977. He called for a new medical model that would integrate biological, psychological, and social mechanisms in order to avoid reductionism. His objective was to challenge the biologism that dominated medicine and health. Engel (1977, 1981) explicitly argued for a model that was holistic and non-reductionistic. Engel's model – based on General Systems Theory (von Bertalanffy, 1973) – was underpinned by an ontology that was arguably similar to critical realism in that it presupposed an emergent, multi-levelled reality.

Critique of the biopsychosocial model

There are two types of critique about the *biopsychosocial* approach: one focusing on its theoretical aspects; and the other on its clinical usefulness. The first type of critique is articulated for example by Weiner (1994) who argues that the model does not fully recognize the complexity of the process of integration of information from different systems. The second type of critique, which is more common, focuses on the model's problems from the viewpoint of a practitioner. For example, Sadler and Hulgus (1990, 1992) argue that the model cannot be used as a guide in the clinical decision-making process because it does not give clear advice to the clinician. We add a third type of critique in which we argue that the biopsychosocial model lacks a metatheoretical grounding, while it nevertheless remains potentially compatible with critical realism.

Richter (1999) suggests that one way of overcoming the theoretical problems with the model is to "dismantle" it. He argues that "each system is functioning by autonomous operations that separates them from each other" (26). The systems are self-organized and they only refer to processes within their own system; i.e. on this conception there is no interaction between them, a standpoint with which we radically disagree. This view of complex systems was developed by Maturana and Varela (1987) and has been further elaborated by the sociologist Niklas Luhmann (1997). However, the idea that the biopsychosocial model consists of "autopoietic systems" – self-referential systems with no exchange of information between them – runs the risk of throwing out the baby with the bathwater. To the contrary, the critical realist position suggests that while the levels of scale are distinct and cannot be reduced to each other, they nevertheless engage in complex interactions – there is therefore communication between these levels. This interaction can be understood by the analysis of constituting structures, mechanisms, and events (see Chapter 6, where we discuss laminated systems). An obvious example of the "communication" between different systems is the previously discussed placebo effect, i.e. there are interaction and exchange of information between the psychological level and the biological level.

The second type of critique of the biopsychosocial model's shortcomings relates to questions of how possible it is for the model to be applied in clinical practice. Underlying this question is the more general issue of translational research – also referred to as translational science – defined by the European Society for Translational Medicine (EUSTM) as "*an interdisciplinary branch of the biomedical field supported by three main pillars: benchside, bedside and community*" (Cohrs et al., 2015: 86; italics in original). According to Cohrs et al., translational medicine and hence translational research form a highly interdisciplinary field, the primary goal being to coalesce assets of various natures within the individual pillars in order to improve the global health care system. When trying to "translate" biopsychosocial research findings into practice in order to achieve meaningful health outcomes, one must bear in mind that there is no straightforward relation between a theoretical model, like the biopsychosocial model, and an individual clinician's decision-making in a face-to-face interaction with a patient. The discussion here is related to a point that we made when outlining the seven enigmas of healing in Chapter 10, which is that interdisciplinary, multimechanism theories are universal transfactuals and there can never be a one-to-one relationship between a universal transfactual and an empirical event (the actual case faced by a clinician) because mediations are unavoidable in the open system of the world. Since a lone clinician is unlikely to have all the knowledge necessary to proceed in a fully interdisciplinary way, interdisciplinarity is likely to require the presence of multi-professional teams and rehabilitation chains. These allow interventions to be co-ordinated from different fields such as medicine, social work, and education.

A critical realist critique of the biopsychosocial model

One reason for the failure of the biopsychosocial model to achieve interdisciplinarity is that practitioners from different fields of health research are likely to have different views on causation. In order to prevent illness, or intervene so as to promote recovery, one needs an understanding of what has brought the manifested illness into being. In both epidemiology and case studies, causality is a "pertinacious question" (Karhausen, 2000). In health research generally there are two dominating perspectives on causality: the "mechanism approach" advocated here; and the "black box" approach (in psychology, the "black box" approach is famously associated with the work of B. F. Skinner [1904–1990]). The first approach involves the idea that phenomena occur because there are mechanisms that produce them and that the aim of research is to reveal these underlying mechanisms. The second approach involves the idea that research should focus on the empirical input and output, and that it is not necessary to conjecture about the internal mechanisms. Indeed, drawing on the philosopher David Hume, some go so far as to argue that the idea of causation can be separated from explanation. For instance, we have known for a long time that smoking increases the probability of lung cancer, but we have not been able to explain this relation until recently.

The mechanism approach is the critical realist approach and it assumes the existence of a structured, emergent ontology. Beyond our empirical observations there are mechanisms that have the properties of producing phenomena, e.g. beyond our observations of falling items there is a mechanism called gravity. The black box approach assumes a flat ontology, and that science is concerned merely with the registration of empirical regularities.

We have throughout this book argued that the mechanism approach is a precondition for interdisciplinarity. The black box approach depends on an inadequate, actualistic view of science which inevitably results in a reductionism of some sort, that is, it results in monodisciplinarity. The consequence of actualism and reductionism is that interdisciplinarity is either unnecessary or impossible. But for many practitioners this reductionism does not fit their reality. In their practice, they encounter human beings, not bodies. The mechanism approach requires an understanding that individual human beings are products-in-process, that is, they are products of their past but they are also in the process of making their future. It requires that we think more deeply about their social and environmental context (space and time) and that we see a human being as a necessarily laminated system. In this way, we can underlabour for translational research (provide it with an adequate metatheoretical base) and overcome the critique that the biopsychosocial model is not useful in practice. We will now take further steps to understand applied interdisciplinary health research by focusing on the ICF.

The ICF

The ICF is widely used as an interdisciplinary way to approach health and wellbeing issues. In this section, we consider the ICF in critical realism terms, in order to propose how the ICF can be further developed. We therefore aim to underlabour for the ICF in pursuit of the first of its four goals: to provide a scientific basis for understanding and studying health and health-related states, outcomes, and determinants.

The general schema of the ICF is illustrated in Figure 11.1. It links (a) health conditions, disorders, or diseases to (b) bodily functions and structures, activities, and participation, and then relates all of these to (c) both environmental and personal factors. The forerunner of the ICF was the International Classification of Impairment, Disability and Handicap in 1980 (ICIDH). In the ICIDH, there were three central concepts – impairment, disability, and handicap. On the one hand,

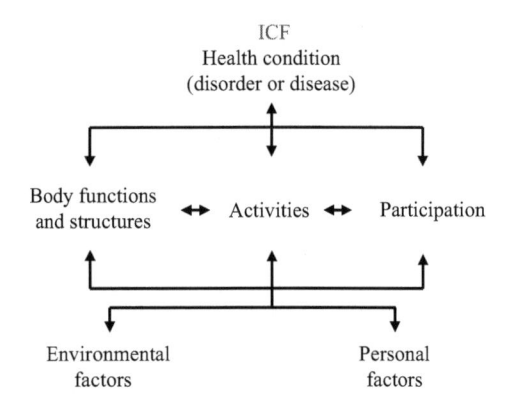

FIGURE 11.1 The biopsychosocial framework of the ICF

the ICIDH focused on the individual and, on the other hand, on the physical disease or impairments. In other words, it was a reductionist, linear approach and therefore the World Health Organization (WHO) decided to reform it, resulting in it being superseded, in 2001, by the ICF.

In the ICF, the state of an individual's health is defined in terms of sets of domains of functioning and disability. These are then evaluated in terms of decreasing function. Each functioning domain interacts with other domains and is multidimensional. For instance, a mild problem with hearing (the functioning domain) is due to multifaceted interactions between intrinsic characteristics of the person (their impairments or limitations) and aspects of their physical, social, and cultural context. Therefore, a multimechanism-based, explanatory framework is necessary in order to appreciate the complexity of the interacting processes that generate the functioning domain. The absence of such a framework will result in reductive, narrow, and linear explanations.

We argue that the ICF is, to date, the most adequate version of Engel's biopsychosocial model, and Bronfenbrenner's Bio-Ecological Systems Theory (Bruyère, VanLooy and Peterson, 2005). It provides an excellent scaffolding of biological, environmental, and social (contextual) information and gives clear advice as to what kinds of data need to be collected and how to usefully combine this data in order to do justice to the biopsychosocial model. It provides useful guidance on how to manipulate and model the data, and how to analyse it. However, the ICF does not purport to contain a metatheoretically grounded conceptual framework. In their attempt to avoid reductionism and linear causality, the designers of the ICF shunned the discussion of causal relationships altogether (Bickenbach et al., 1999). It is therefore merely a taxonomy or list based on what is known empirically. Furthermore, it does not provide the intellectual tools required to integrate the information obtained by using it. Because the ICF does not a priori suggest causal connections between the various components of the models, and therefore the various sets of data, it is compatible with a range of theoretical explanations. It thus avoids reductive knowledge, but does this by avoiding theories altogether. Some argue (e.g. Imrie, 2004) that as a consequence the ICF is underdetermined from a theoretical perspective. We agree that the ICF lacks theory, but this does not prevent it from being used as the basis to develop such theory. Significantly, the ICF sets the stage for interdisciplinarity by insisting on multidisciplinarity. This is because, when using the ICF, one cannot code the magnitude of a disability in a domain without also considering the context and the way that the domain may hinder a person's participation. Specifically, the basic content required by interdisciplinary health researchers and practitioners – provided by the ICF – includes: (a) a biological-level model that addresses the causal links between body functions and structures; (b) a person-level model that considers the person's basic activities; and (c) a context-level model that links the body and the person's activities to their overall context (Stucki et al., 2007; Stucki and Grimby, 2007). The ICF therefore provides the basic multidisciplinary grounds for epistemic novelty that is a condition of interdisciplinary research. In other words, it provides a good basis for retroductive theorizing about real causal mechanisms and structures.

Nevertheless, while the ICF provides the groundwork for interdisciplinarity, on its own it merely achieves multidisciplinarity since it avoids theory about structures and mechanisms. Therefore, it depends on the researchers who use it to take it to the level of interdisciplinarity. Not all researchers are interested to take this next step, or have the philosophical tools to do so, tools that we trust we are providing in this book.

The principal exponents of the ICF approach are Gerold Stucki et al. (2007). They offer a powerful critique of the monodisciplinary, biomedical perspective to human function. In many respects their work is exemplary and we fully endorse their advocacy of interdisciplinary thinking in relation to health and wellbeing. Indeed, their approach arguably has many commonalities with critical realism, for instance it is explicitly based on a "level ontology" (from cell to society, 666). Stucki et al. (2007) provide a broad, widely inclusive framework that includes more than immediate socio-economic issues, but also human development, philosophy, history, ethics, and public health, amongst other things. In dealing with rehabilitation, they suggest that research should be categorized into three types of science, namely:

i   basic science: the fields of human functioning science and biosciences in rehabilitation;
ii applied science: the fields of integrative rehabilitation science and biomedical rehabilitation science and engineering; and
iii professional sciences: the field of professional rehabilitation sciences.

However, their work would benefit from an adequate metatheory in order to be able to thematize ontology. By not addressing the basic questions related to ontology and by focusing on epistemology, Stucki et al. (2007) can only suggest educational and organizational/professional solutions to the problem of monodisciplinarity, such as broader academic training programmes and increased career, publishing, and funding opportunities (see Table 2.1). The absence of metatheory also results in the absence of an in-depth discussion of the crucial phase of interdisciplinary research in which scientists integrate their knowledge from the five proposed scientific fields into a holistic understanding of the human being. Like Stucki et al., we agree that there is a need for specialization and division of labour in the field of human functioning and rehabilitation research. However, the challenge is to integrate this knowledge. In other words, the useful suggestions made by Stucki et al. (2007) – designed to make human functioning and rehabilitation research truly interdisciplinary – can only be operationalized if they are underpinned by a metatheory of the sort advocated here.

ICF core sets

For many, the holistic approach adopted by the WHO and reflected in the ICF was a welcome relief from the reductionism that dominated the field of health and human functioning. However, the use of the ICF schema in practice has proven cumbersome. It has 1,454 items in its schema, which is designed to be comprehensive and thus to include every disorder, disease, and disability. These items relate to such things as a person's ability to manage daily routines, to acquire complex skills, and to produce nonverbal messages; and they are divided into *core sets* in order to simplify the classification system and to make it more manageable in general practice. These core sets specify the most important factors or influences related to specific health conditions as described earlier, drawn from all five constituent aspects, namely, bodily structure and functions, activities, participation, environmental factors, and personal factors. The core sets come in three forms: comprehensive, brief, and generic:

- The Comprehensive ICF Core Set covers the entire spectrum of typical problems faced by people with a particular health condition. It provides a thorough and interdisciplinary checklist to prevent practitioners from overlooking aspects of a patient's functioning.
- The Brief ICF Core Set includes categories derived from the Comprehensive ICF Core Set that capture the essence of a person's experience of functioning and disability. It is used when only a brief assessment of functioning is necessary.
- The Generic Set consists of seven ICF categories that best differentiate the different levels of functioning among persons with any health condition. The Generic Set is used to compare functioning across health conditions, settings, contexts, countries, and population groups.

The consensual process of developing core sets follows a set procedure outlined in Figure 11.2. In the preparatory phase, studies are conducted from the perspectives of the researchers, patients, experts, and clinicians, respectively. Then, in Phase I, there is a conference oriented to the establishment of a consensus of the most important items in the ICF covering a particular condition, such as hearing loss (Delbeq, Van de Ven and Gustafson, 1975). For each condition, the number of items is reduced to a more manageable number, about 50 or 60 items, out of the more than 1,400 defined in the ICF's comprehensive scheme. In Phase II, these core sets are subject to a number of field tests in different parts of the world.

The ICF is based on the ontology of empirical realism – it therefore collapses three levels of reality (real, actual, empirical) into one (empirical). Therefore, although a core set is multidisciplinary and thus reflects different areas of functioning, it is not the same as a laminated system in the critical realist sense because it considers these different areas only in terms of the empirical evidence, and not what this empirical evidence tells us about the deeper levels of reality of structures and mechanisms that are not empirical. A good core set therefore describes the most significant features of a health issue on the empirical surface of reality but it does not provide the generative mechanisms or causal structures that produce a particular kind of phenomenon or type of effect. A consequence is that the core sets are not anchored by a deep, transfactual theory that shows the mechanisms at work.

120 Applied interdisciplinary research

```
    Preparatory Phase              Phase I                  Phase

┌─────────────────────────┐  ┌──────────────────┐   ┌──────────────────┐
│ Researcher perspective  │  │                  │   │                  │
│ (Systematic review)     │  │  ICF Core Sets   │   │                  │
│                         │  │    Consensus     │   │     Testing      │
│                         │  │    Conference    │   │       of         │
│ Patient perspective     │  │                  │   │ the ICF Core Sets│
│ (Qualitative study)     │  │        ⇩         │   │                  │
│                         │  │                  │   │                  │
│ Expert perspective      │  │   1st version of │   │                  │
│ (Expert survey)         │  │  the ICF Core Sets│  │                  │
│                         │  │                  │   │                  │
│ Clinical perspective    │  │                  │   │                  │
│ (Cross-sectional study) │  │                  │   │                  │
└─────────────────────────┘  └──────────────────┘   └──────────────────┘

       Year 1                     Year 2                 Year 3
```

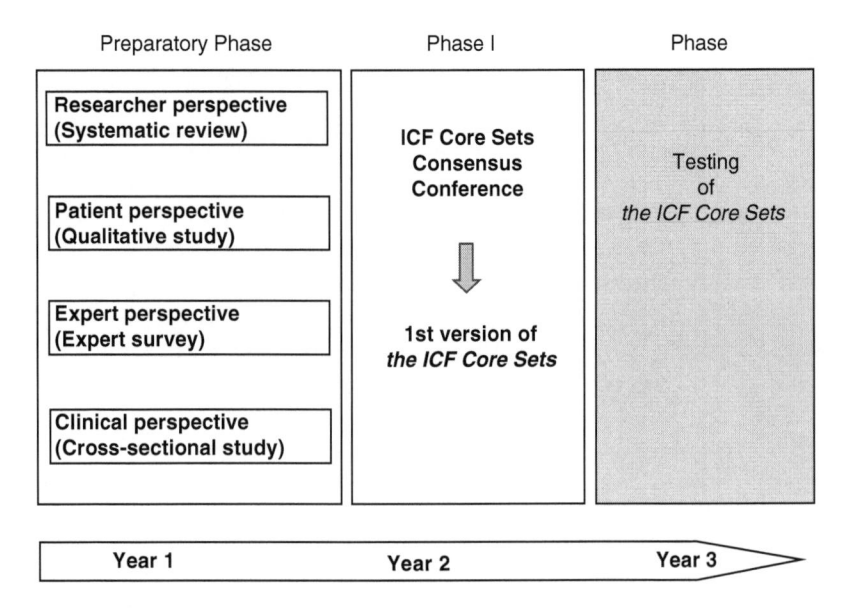

FIGURE 11.2 The phases in the development of the ICF core sets

There are at least two ways that an empiricist realist might try to make up for the absence of transfactual theory to explain a functional challenge. First, they might attempt to record every empirical piece of evidence of the functional challenge. This results in an overload of information; and it is not reliable information because it is easily challenged by different circumstances, due to the open system of the world (the problem of induction) (Chapter 8). Second, they might turn to expert or first-hand knowledge, or consensus. However, this arguably merely displaces transfactual knowledge about a condition elsewhere (onto the contributors and participants at ICF workshops) and veils its presence, since those contributing to the ICF core sets are likely to bring to the table their transfactual, theoretical knowledge of the condition. This also suggests that the ICF is a TINA compromise (cf. Chapter 7) since, despite its stated claim to eschew theory, its success may be largely due to its ability to smuggle ideologically-based theories of functioning into the consensus-making process. These two issues are reflected in two well-established criticisms of the ICF, namely that it is unwieldy to use because it is based on, and requires, large amounts of empirical data; and that it is theoretically underdetermined.

The critical realist solution to these problems is the concrete universal/singular (cf. Chapter 7, step 3). If we try to apply the concept of the concrete universal/singular to the core sets for hearing loss, then every person with hearing loss (PHL) will contain four aspects, which are:

1. Every PHL is a universal PHL (concrete universal)

    In virtue of being a PHL – in virtue of the real structures and mechanisms that result in her condition, that we know by the epistemological process of transdisciplinarity – she will have certain characteristics in common with all other PHL.

2. Every PHL is a mediated PHL

    Nevertheless, in virtue of being a PHL, she will also have certain characteristics in common with some but not all other PHL. These are her mediations, or her specificities.

3. Every PHL has a geo-historical trajectory

    All PHL come from different space times; they all have a different trajectory. The PHL in question may come from Norway, China, Nepal, or the USA and each of these places will have different cultural ways of supporting (or discriminating against) PHL. However, the trajectory of the PHL is not just geographical, it is also historical, because PHL are born at different times, and therefore a PHL born today may have significantly different life opportunities compared to 50 years ago, resulting in significantly different loss of functioning.

4. Every PHL is a unique individual (concrete singular)

    Even if two PHL came from exactly the same place and were born at the same time, they would not be same because of many other mediating factors, from genetics to family structure, and this results in concrete singularity, or irreducible uniqueness.

Point 1 in the preceding list, the universal characteristics, would be a good basis for the Brief ICF Core Set for hearing loss; and all the four points together (that is, the combination of universal and singular characteristics) would be a good basis for the Comprehensive ICF Core Set for hearing loss. The Generic ICF Core Set would be, from a critical realist perspective, based on a different concrete universal altogether – the set of all people with disabilities (instead of the set of all people with hearing loss). In this case, a patient's actual health challenge (such as hearing loss) would be one of the mediations resulting in her status as a unique concrete singular. She would nevertheless also be a concrete universal who reflects the problems faced by all people with health issues. When classifying a person with hearing loss, one would also need to consider the purpose of the classification (cf. the transitive dimension, Chapter 4). To some extent, this flexibility is provided by the ICF, since one can choose whether to use the Generic or Comprehensive Core Sets, depending on whether one is making a classification simply for administrative purposes, or for medical intervention purposes.

In its current formulation, a problematic consequence of the use of the consensus approach by the ICF to determine the core sets is that biomedical aspects are privileged over socio-economic aspects. This is because it is in practice easier to reach a consensus over biomedical factors than socioeconomic factors. For instance, Scott-Samuel et al. (2014) claim that the worldwide trend towards the commercialization of the health sector has negatively affected service delivery in the health sector. However, most governments disagree and argue that privatization brings significant benefit (Organisation for Economic Co-operation and Development, 2010). This reflects the existence of conflicting interests in society; and the result is that the effects of commercialization (a socio-economic factor) have tended to be underplayed. This is an example of how a TINA compromise is maintained in practice. In this case, the false epistemology – that we can adequately categorize health issues without theoretically understanding the interdisciplinary structures and mechanisms that lead to them – is kept in place because it maintains the dominant status of certain institutions (the biomedical industries who can then monopolize the field and the governments who can then avoid criticism of their socio-economic policy) (cf. Chapter 5). In Chapter 13, we saw how certain groups can maintain their power by determining the content of communication media. In this case, powerful biomedical groups can insist on a primarily biomedical content of the ICF by ensuring that their representatives form a majority of the participants at the conferences for the development of the ICF core sets. If we agree that the difference between democracy and populism is the presence or absence of civil education and the voting population's access to objective information, then encouraging a critical realist version (that is, not a Humean version) of objectivity to decide interdisciplinary health issues would benefit a democratic approach to the core sets. Critical realist objectivity is one that is based on judgemental rationality, rather than empiricist scientific method. This means that a consensus approach would still be necessary, but only after a thoroughly scientific and interdisciplinary treatment of the issues had been undertaken, accompanied by a transparent process of choosing, by judgemental rationality, transfactual theory to explain the evidence. Such transparency would potentially uncover attempts to choose a theory that suits certain agendas, rather than one that best explains all the evidence (no matter how inconvenient this truth may be to certain sectors of society). Ontologically speaking, biomedical causes do not have greater importance than other causes. It simply already is the case that other causes are at play, such as psychological and social causes, whether socio-economic or cultural. It is also the case that the longer we take to understand the aetiology of a condition, the more pressing will be the need to account for the non-biomedical causes – the psychosocial causes – such as behaviour and lifestyle.

In this chapter, we explored the idea of the biopsychosocial approach to understanding health and wellbeing, and we constructively critiqued one example of the utilization of the concept, the ICF. While we argued that both the concept of the biopsychosocial approach, and its manifestation in the ICF, are extremely useful first steps towards interdisciplinarity, we also argued they are unable to achieve interdisciplinarity because they are hampered by a flat, Humean ontology (black box approach). We suggested that instead they need to acknowledge that ontology is layered and emergent. This will allow them to theorize the existence of transfactual, universal structures and mechanisms. While universal structures and mechanisms are always mediated by the open system of the world, and therefore there is never a one-to-one manifestation of them in practice, nevertheless they exist and we can know about them.

12

THE PRACTICAL ORGANIZATION OF INTERDISCIPLINARY CO-OPERATION

In this chapter, we use the framework of critical realist metatheory to consider in more detail the requirements of interdisciplinary co-operation and dialogue. We do this by outlining the temporal logic of interdisciplinary research and by considering the differences between reductionist, atomist, and integrated approaches to health and wellbeing. We explain why interdisciplinarity requires, rather than avoids, disciplinary specialization. We also offer a brief overview and critique of the available literature's solutions to the problem of interdisciplinarity.

We have argued that interdisciplinary research is based on the assumption that the real intransitive object of inquiry is always-already unified, complex, and emergent. It cannot be otherwise. However, the fragmentation of the sciences as currently constituted makes it difficult to arrive at knowledge that reflects this unified, complex, and emergent reality. While some differentiation and specialization (monodisciplinarity) in health and wellbeing research are not only unavoidable but also beneficial, nevertheless, we also need a degree of unity in order to reach integration and holistic understanding. It is unity-in-difference that we are seeking, but the problem is that there is often a mismatch between the disciplines and the unified objects that they study. In other words, we have a unified object that exists at different, emergent levels of reality but current approaches to interdisciplinarity provide a fragmented understanding of it. To achieve integration, that is, to achieve true interdisciplinarity, the multidisciplinary research team must move beyond the empirical to develop transfactual theories of the real multimechanisms at play at every emergent level.

In Figure 12.1 we outline the temporal logic of interdisciplinary research (see also Chapter 6). The different phases are analytical in the sense that they rarely exist in a pure way. Rather, they tend to overlap and researchers will often move back and forth between them. To begin with, we broach the research topic through the individual disciplines, in a broadly reductive moment. We then move into the multidisciplinary phase which requires crossdisciplinary understanding. After this, we are able to achieve interdisciplinarity through retroductive transdisciplinary explanatory theorizing about the structures and mechanisms at the level of the emergent real. Epistemic emergence is the creative process by which new, transdisciplinary knowledge is achieved from a multidisciplinary groundwork. Although Figure 12.1 is designed from the perspective of team work, nevertheless, transdisciplinary theorizing can also be carried out by multidisciplinary-minded individuals.

We can see from Figure 12.1 that the objective of an interdisciplinary research team is to achieve an integrated knowledge of an (always-already integrated) intransitive object. Thus we go from an initial state t_0 in which, at the epistemological level, disciplines are completely split, each pursuing effectively a reductionist approach. This phase is necessary; one can say that it is a precondition for success in the other phases. In order to successfully contribute to an interdisciplinary team, one has first to be a skilled and experienced disciplinary researcher.

We progress at t_1 to the multidisciplinary phase of research in which the different disciplines are aware of the need to utilize the insights of the others in a full explanation of the phenomena. However, this phase does not yet provide the synthetic integrated knowledge which would be adequate to the (already

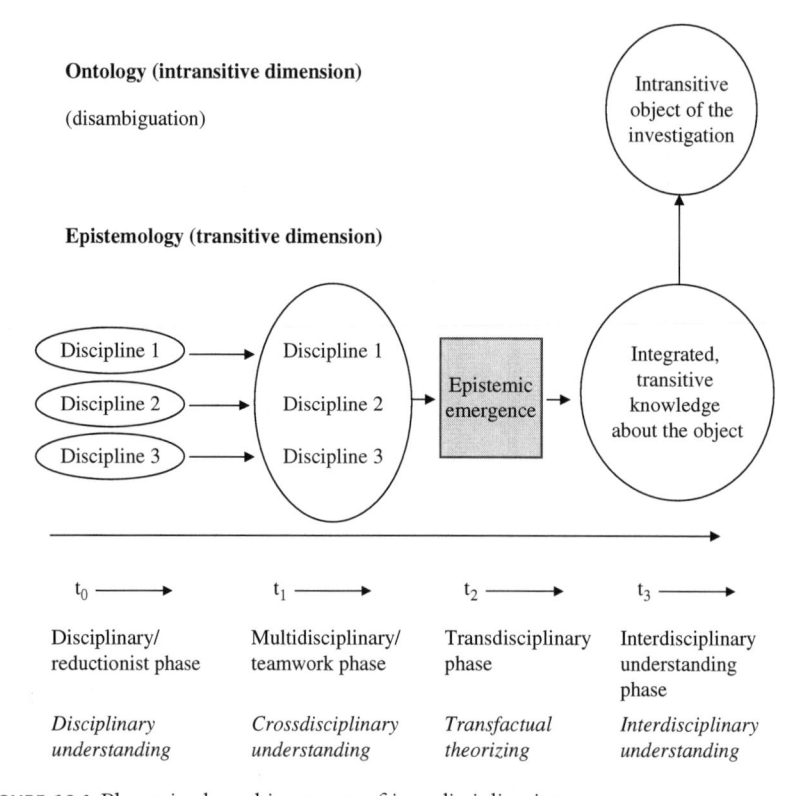

FIGURE 12.1 Phases in the achievement of interdisciplinarity

integrated) intransitive object. This phase – the multidisciplinary phase – involves crossdisciplinary understanding. The implication of this cannot be underestimated. It includes learning from other disciplines or areas of knowledge. By learning from other researchers one increases the possibilities of creative solutions. In this phase a number of challenges occur. One of the most important is the question of respect for other disciplines. Knowledge of other disciplines lays the foundation for understanding them, which in turn leads to respect for their practitioners. Lack of recognition and respect of others in the team is devastating for the next phase.

To get to the final stage, t_3, of an interdisciplinary, integrated understanding of the intransitive object of investigation, we need to go through phase t_2 of transdisciplinarity. This is the stage of epistemic emergence and transfactual theorizing. If the researchers remain at t_0, their research will become reductionist. If they remain at t_1, their research will become atomist. At t_2 the epistemic emergence may be the result of retroduction or retrodiction, or a combination of the two. Note that this model of interdisciplinarity is valid for answering both concrete universal questions, such as "What causes it?" or "What heals it?" and concrete singular questions, such as "How can we heal it, in this case?" It can be used by a multidisciplinary team of medical researchers in a laboratory, exploring a concrete universal (e.g. the universal disease of diabetes), or by a multidisciplinary team of medical practitioners in a hospital setting, dealing with the concrete singulars of their actual cases (individual people, each uniquely expressing, due to mediations, the universal disease of diabetes).

From a metatheoretical perspective, the problem is that the human being is a laminated totality (in the ontological dimension, as represented by four-planar social being in Figure 5.1). As such, an adequate explanation cannot be achieved by either a reductionist perspective (reducing our understanding of an individual to a part or parts of the individual) or an atomistic perspective (claiming that any one of the biological, psychological, or social aspects can be understood in isolation from the other two aspects). To illustrate the difference between reductionism and atomism, and to compare these to an integrated approach, we will use the example of Attention Deficit Hyperactivity Disorder (ADHD):

- A practitioner with a biologically reductionist view might assume that we can fully explain ADHD in terms of a chemical imbalance in the brain and thus simply prescribe Ritalin. If they have a behaviourally reductionist view, they might see the problem as one of behaviour and simply prescribe an occupational therapist. Another version of reductionism might be social constructionism. In this case, the practitioner might deny that ADHD is a real condition and prefer to see it as a socially constructed entity that can simply be avoided by changing the way that society perceives normal behaviour.
- A practitioner with an atomistic view of ADHD might agree that there are several mechanisms at different levels which contribute to, or shape, the

phenomenon, but they would fail to consider the interplay of these mechanisms. They might try to deal broadly with the different levels of reality of the ADHD person's life, for example, they might prescribe behaviour change therapies, while also suggesting the use of Ritalin to address the chemical imbalance, and attempting to address problems associated with the negative social construction of the disease.

- A practitioner with an integrated view of ADHD will have a transdisciplinary, transfactual theory about ADHD that will help to make sense of the condition at each of the levels of reality. For instance, one such transfactual theory is known as the neurodiversity theory (Bhandari and Khanal, 2016; Jaarsma and Welin, 2012). It suggests that human beings do not have only one genetically stamped mental mode of being that is normal, but several, each with evolutionarily adaptive or maladaptive consequences (depending on context and the degree of phenotypic expression of the condition):

Thus *autism* is associated with computational careers, *depression* with literary creativity, *schizophrenia* with lateral thinking and the Odyssean personality, *ADHD* with an Ice-Age readiness to respond, *obsessive compulsive disorder* with a focused range of interests, and *Tourette's syndrome* with competitive sports and jazz improvisation.

(Bradshaw and Sheppard, 2000: 297, italics in original; see also Crawford and Salmon, 2004)

This theory is relevant to all the levels of the understanding of ADHD, that is, it integrates the genetic, the social, the economic, and the behavioural aspects of it. Because of this transfactual knowledge, the integrated practitioner will understand how the different levels of the issue interact. They will perhaps realize that, while the use of behaviour-change therapies and medication may sometimes be helpful, at other times such interventions may impede the person's other abilities and that it may not always be in the best interests of the person's or society's overall flourishing to insist on "normal" integration. Medication may therefore not be the best option for all ADHD patients, depending on their level of disability and the degree to which their ADHD is adaptive to their life-world and personal life objectives. The integrated approach might therefore include steps to support individuals to develop their special talents, while at the same time not denying the role that medication and social-coping skills can play.

An important reason behind reductionism is the contemporary approach to specialization in the health care system. Specialization allows our knowledge to deepen, but without an understanding that reality is layered, and therefore, without the integrating aspect of transfactual knowledge of structures and mechanisms, this knowledge remains disjointed. From the perspective of an empiricist, this process results in an epistemic paradox, as the more knowledge that they gain of the parts of the individual, the more that they realize they do not know about how these parts interact. The empiricists' ontology and epistemology leave them with no way to overcome this paradox. For critical realists, however, specialization is an important aspect of the scientific method, but only initially. For instance, it is included in the RRREI(C) in terms of the second R, which refers to the Resolution of the issue into its component parts. A practical consequence of this intuitively derived truth about epistemology is that the health care system has become organized by specialisms at different levels of reality, namely at the levels of the biological, psychological, and social. However, when these specialisms are not re-integrated through the process of transfactual theorizing (the third R, i.e. Retrodiction), then there are a number of negative consequences. For instance, patients experience the need for specialists of various sorts, yet these specialists often do not interact and for the most part are ignorant of each other and their subject matters, or laboratory researchers work in isolation on aspects of a disease without communicating with field researchers and epidemiologists. Currently, the dominant epistemology, of empiricism, results in the assumption that empirical knowledge exhausts reality. Therefore, specialists are skilled at describing and treating the empirical symptoms of their own specialism but find it hard to move beyond this because they are not provided with the epistemological tools to do so. However, if they were to have a critical realist epistemology, one which acknowledged the reality of emergent realms, and one which had a multimechanism view of causality, then they would have an epistemological justification for embarking on interdisciplinary co-operation in order to gain an understanding (through transfactual theories and categories) of the emergent levels of ontological reality of which their particular specializations are a part. In other words, to avoid a fragmented health care outcome, it is necessary not only to move beyond linear causality (reductionism and monodisciplinarity), but also to move beyond multi-causality (atomism and multidisciplinarity). We can achieve this through retroductive theorizing (transdisciplinarity) about transfactual multimechanism reality, which results in interdisciplinarity.

Therefore, the search for interdisciplinarity does not mean giving up one's speciality. In the leap from multidisciplinarity to interdisciplinarity, the disciplines are not collapsed, but enhanced. This is because the emergent orders of reality cannot be reduced to the lower orders. These must be studied as entities in their own right. For example, it would be impossible to understand how a genetic problem causes a disease without having an excellent understanding of chemistry. It would be impossible to consider the psychological problems facing a recent amputee without having an excellent understanding of the biological and physical constraints that their disability places on them. Therefore, this approach does not discourage specialization, but may even enhance it, as the various specialisms are integrated into a coherent totality, which is more than the sum of its parts. The coherent totality does not result in the collapse of the levels and mechanisms, but puts them into a context where their efficacy can be displayed. Specialization is here to stay, but it cannot be accompanied by isolation. At present, we have a large amount of knowledge about the details of various health-related mechanisms. The challenge is to increase our understanding of the variety of holistic situations in which these mechanisms interact and to understand how these mechanisms are themselves emergent. Next we will consider how someone with a strong disciplinary grounding might be supported to work well in an interdisciplinary team.

In interdisciplinary team work, as we have suggested (see Table 2.1), there are a number of barriers to successful cooperation. In Table 12.1, we outline the main recommendations in the literature on how to overcome these barriers, referring mainly (but not exclusively) to those made by leading international research organizations. These include: the European Union Research Advisory Board (EURAB-EU); National Academy of Sciences (NAS-USA); National Academy of Engineering (USA); and Institute of Medicine (USA) (for further details see EURAB, 2004: 1; NAS, 2004: 110–113). For each recommendation we give some examples of concrete activity that might support it.

Another useful outline of the types of mechanisms that can support interdisciplinarity is provided by Rowe (2008: 5–7). He divides these mechanisms into three groups: investigator-specific, project-specific, and external factors. The first group of investigator-specific factors includes:

- passion for the work and true openness to the approach, perspectives, and attitudes of scientists from other disciplines;
- mutual respect of scientists in the team;
- complementary skills and knowledge;
- ability of scientists to develop a common language; and
- ability to meet together on a regular basis.

The second group of factors includes: data sources such as longitudinal samples and established research populations; new integrative concepts; and emergence of new technologies. The third group of factors is external and includes: funding; institutional flexibility and freedom; career advancement issues; and attitudes towards interdisciplinary research.

Both the recommendations by Rowe (2008), and those summarized in Table 12.1, provide practical advice on achieving interdisciplinarity. However, not much is said about the metatheoretical and theoretical aspects of interdisciplinary research. Therefore, these recommendations mainly address the problems at the lower level of the initial list in Table 2.1. Nevertheless, the need for metatheoretical unity is hinted at when Rowe (2008) suggests: (a) the need to provide opportunities to learn from other disciplines; and (b) the need to establish agreements about research methods at an early stage. As we suggested in Chapter 2 (Table 2.1), in order to learn from other disciplines and to agree on research methods, it is necessary to establish a common metatheoretical approach, such as is provided by critical realism. It is only within such an approach that one can anchor an agreement about methods.

Therefore, as laudable as these recommendations are, they cannot by themselves lead the research team towards interdisciplinary integration. However, some might argue that disciplinary differences (and here they might include epistemological and ontological differences) are an important driving force for the team members to

TABLE 12.1 Recommendations from the literature for successful interdisciplinarity

Recommendations	Examples
Academic institutions should develop and strengthen existing policies and practices that lower or remove barriers to interdisciplinary research and scholarship, including developing joint programmes with industry and government and nongovernment organizations (NAS); and avoiding unnecessary administrative barriers to interdisciplinarity (EURAB)	– Establish interdisciplinary review committees to evaluate faculty who are conducting interdisciplinarity – Give high priority to recruitment of researchers whose focus is interdisciplinary – Develop policy that insists that interdisciplinary teams include researchers from the social sciences and humanities
Institutions should experiment with more innovative policies and structures to facilitate interdisciplinarity, making appropriate use of lessons from the performance of interdisciplinarity in industrial and national laboratories (NAS); interdisciplinary centres should be established (EURAB)	– Ensure that the centre has made provision for interdisciplinarity within the teaching and research activities of the traditional disciplinary departments – Experiment with alternatives to departmental tenure through new modes of employment, retention, and promotion – Create mechanisms to fund graduate students and postdoctoral scholars whose research draws on multiple fields and may not be considered central to any one department
Institutions should support interdisciplinary education and training for students, postdoctoral scholars, researchers, and faculty by providing such mechanisms as undergraduate research opportunities, faculty team-teaching credit, and the management of interdisciplinary training (NAS); improve current interdisciplinary training (EURAB)	– Support formal programmes on the management of interdisciplinary programmes, including leadership and team-forming activities – Develop graduate school structures which, when required, can more easily span traditional disciplinary divisions in research training – Provide opportunities (such as sabbaticals) for students and faculty members to learn the content, languages, and cultures of disciplines other than their own, both within and outside their home institution
Institutions should develop equitable and flexible budgetary and cost-sharing policies that support interdisciplinarity (NAS); institutions should share research facilities; funds should be specifically available for interdisciplinarity (EURAB)	– Streamline fair and equitable budgeting procedures across department or school lines to allocate resources to interdisciplinary units outside the departments or schools – Ensure that the structuring of work programme budgets does not discriminate against interdisciplinary projects
To facilitate the work of an interdisciplinary team, its leaders should bring together potential research collaborators early in the process and work towards agreement on key issues (NAS); there should be clear procedures for managing interdisciplinarity (EURAB)	– Encourage integrated designs of research proposals rather than "stapling together" similar or overlapping proposals – Establish agreements on research methods, goals, and timelines at an early stage – Have regular interdisciplinary meetings
Interdisciplinary team leaders should seek to ensure that each participant strikes an appropriate balance between leading and following and between contributing to and benefiting from the efforts of the team (NAS)	– Provide adequate time for mutual learning – Help the team to decide who will be responsible for each portion of the research plan

sharpen their positions and arguments and hence further develop in their disciplines and that at the end of the day the outcome of the research would benefit from the differences. We agree that arguments, differences, and conflicts are important and valuable parts of coming to interdisciplinary understanding. However, these will remain unresolved if there is no common metatheoretical ground upon which to base them. In other words, if epistemological consensus is not reached – regarding for instance disambiguation of ontology and epistemology, explicit non-reductionism, or the idea of a laminated system – then the most important phase of the research, the integration of knowledge into a broader understanding, will be hampered. A number of case studies have provided strong empirical support to our argument that such ontological and epistemological consensus is vital to the success of interdisciplinarity (see e.g. Sawa, 2005; Pohl, 2005; Stokols et al., 2005).

Interdisciplinarity is part of a process that builds on disciplinarity and multidisciplinarity. Our objective as health practitioners is to avoid the reductionism and atomism that occur when we fail to follow through to interdisciplinary understanding via transdisciplinary theorizing about emergent structures and mechanisms at the level of the real. A key component of interdisciplinary co-operation is respect for disciplines other than our own. This brings us to the question of why such respect is so difficult to achieve, related to the question of disciplinary imperialism, which we discuss in the next chapter.

13

UNDERSTANDING METHODOLOGICAL IMPERIALISM

Methodological imperialism is the understanding that some methods or methodologies are considered to be "proper" science, while others are considered to be less scientific or even not scientific at all. In Table 2.1, we mentioned the existence of "methodological imperialism". In this chapter, we attempt to understand its nature and origins and some of the language-based mechanisms by which it is maintained.

Some biomedical scientists assume that qualitative methods do not generate valid knowledge because these methods are not based on the experimental canon (Albert et al., 2008). However, this attitude reflects ignorance amongst the biomedical practitioners. First, ignorance about what characterizes qualitative methods, i.e. methodological ignorance (qualitative, non-experimental methods can generate valid knowledge). Second, ignorance about what constitutes scientific research, i.e. epistemological ignorance (qualitative, non-experimental methods are scientific). Third, ignorance about ontology, i.e. ontological ignorance (ontology is not exhausted by the empirical level of reality, and knowledge about real, non-empirical ontological structures and mechanisms can only be grasped via qualitative methods).

Unfortunately, the qualitative/quantitative hierarchy reported in Albert et al. (2008) is widespread and many, if not all, social scientists have experienced the devaluation of their research that accompanies it (Holland, 2014). However, there are variations of this hierarchy. For instance, a report from the USA's NAS (2004) revealed that most deans and heads of department hold the opinion that interdisciplinary research is not "at the edge of science". Another example of the hierarchy is present in research design communities, where the randomized controlled trial (RCT) is claimed to be "the gold standard" of research, applicable far beyond its original use, i.e. tests of medical treatments. As a result, in-depth case studies are considered to be less scientifically sound and therefore less valuable. Our argument is not to detract from the different and important question of what constitutes good and bad science; nevertheless, it is incorrect to equate quantitative, monodisciplinary, or experimental science with good science – and qualitative, interdisciplinary, non-experimental science with bad, or lesser, science.

A key to overcoming the hierarchies of the disciplines is to remember that the logic common to all science is retroduction and that this logic is part of a dialectical scientific process summed up by the DREI(C) approach (cf. Chapter 6). This automatically levels the playing field since whether one is a psychologist, a sociologist, or a geneticist one will be acquainted with and able to use the DREI(C). This step towards interdisciplinarity is perhaps mainly a mental transition for most natural scientists since, as we have already explained, their practice has always belied their use of the DREI(C), and it has merely been their self-conscious theoretical reflections that failed to match their actual practice (see also Holland in Price, 2016). Nevertheless, it is still an important mental transition to make as it allows those scientists who were previously placed lower in the disciplinary hierarchy because of their greater engagement with the non-empirical, emergent levels of reality to properly take their place next to those scientists who deal more directly with empirical reality. In other words, it puts the psychologists and the sociologists on the same level as the psychiatrists and the medical doctors. Currently, this is not the case and researchers tend to assume not only incommensurability between their methods and those of other members of an interdisciplinary team, but that the opinions of practitioners whose methods are more empirically based are inherently more valuable. To the contrary, while it is true that in any particular instance, not every specialization should be given equal weight, nevertheless the weight allocated to a specialization should not be determined by the degree to which the specialization is based on the empirical layer of reality. Rather, it should be determined by the special requirements of the context. For example, in one case psychology might be most important (where the health problems are mainly due to non-empirical, emergent mental structures), but in another case, psychiatry might be most important (where the health problems are mainly due to empirical chemical imbalances in the brain), although in either case, both psychiatry and psychology may play a role.

The question that remains is: Why do these hierarchies exist? Due to the emergent, complex nature of ontology, one cannot a priori maintain and rationally justify such hierarchies; they cannot be legitimized with in-depth philosophical and metatheoretical arguments. Hence, there seem to be other mechanisms involved; and we believe that these mechanisms relate to issues of power.

Power and disciplinary hierarchies

Any critical realist discussion of power must first distinguish between what Bhaskar calls power$_1$ and power$_2$. This refers to the distinction between power as transformative capacity (power$_1$) and power as domination or oppression (power$_2$). Such domination is often exercised in the context of master–slave-type relations, a relation that is found at the level of social structure. Second, we wish to distinguish between power *in* representation and power *behind* representation (drawing from Fairclough, 2001; see also Danermark & Germundsson, 2011).

Power in representation

When researchers get together to co-operate on a project, they need to have an articulated representation of what the real world is, around which they can focus their co-operation. Without such a representation, meaningful and successful communication would not be possible. These encounters are sometimes characterized by unequal power, i.e. some participants are more powerful than others and therefore their representations are allocated more weight. If there is conflict, the representations held by the more powerful trump the other, less powerful representations. These inequalities in power stem from the different hierarchies that exist in the scientific community. In order to understand how such relations are constituted and maintained one has to understand the mechanisms influencing the interaction between the researchers. There are at least three ways that a powerful participant can control and constrain the encounter, and so be oppressive (i.e. reflect power$_2$ relations):

- the content of the discussion;
- the relations people enter into, both with respect to each other and any given representation; and
- the subject positions the participants can occupy.

Power over the content may be achieved by the careful selection of information or the careful wording of it. This can mask structural or bureaucratic power relations and present a false picture of harmony, or might support an ideological myth. For example, a powerful individual might hold that a reductionist, medication-based approach to a disease is the accepted approach amongst medical professionals – supporting a particular pharmaceutical brand – when in fact this is not the case and interdisciplinary approaches are in existence and are advocated by some professionals. Controlling the content is often a result of how elaborated a representation is, since the more elaborated it is, the more credence it is given. Because elaboration is *both* a marker of social standing *and* often a more comprehensive picture of the reality in question, its latter advantage may be used as the "innocent" stated justification for it, even if social standing is the main objective. In this way its power$_2$ effects are veiled (Bernstein, 1971). An elaborated description – in the sense of a comprehensive and technical one – should nevertheless be chosen over a competing restricted description if it is rationally justified, but not simply because it is elaborated. That is, we should choose between competing theories of truth according to their ability to fully explain the evidence (judgemental rationality). Actors with *elaborated* but *different* representations arguably have the greatest potential to trigger power mechanisms and to reveal power struggles. For instance, both qualitative and quantitative researchers have elaborated but different codes, and since they are likely to be well-educated and middle class, we can also assume that they expect their knowledge to be taken seriously; this sets the scene for dramatic "science wars" (Price, 2014a). However, also problematic but in a different way is the situation in which one actor is too easily swayed by another because they have a limited, restricted code, and thus perhaps also a lack of confidence in their abilities to distinguish between truth claims. If such an actor is "offered" a description and explanation of some aspects of a phenomenon that (s)he does not fully grasp, (s)he may uncritically accept it wholesale. Hence it must be incumbent upon the interdisciplinary researcher to avoid both the pitfalls of arrogant dismissal of, and fawning assent to, other agents' accounts. Conceivably, a dominant actor with a more elaborated code could take advantage of their $power_1$ to insist on a certain representation that serves their interests ($power_2$). It seems that ethical interdisciplinary behaviour would avoid such $power_2$ play. Instead, the empowered agent might share information with the less powerful agent, while also being open for information to flow both ways, thus potentially empowering both of them, and bringing them into equal $power_1$ standing relative to each other. Refusing to share information is one way to maintain $power_2$, as it results in unequal access to $power_1$. When two different representations result in miscommunication, this may simply be an innocent but unfortunate result of the disciplinary differences, or it may be a calculated means of excluding "outsiders" (Fairclough, 2001: 64).

If two researchers from different professional cultures, such as a psychiatrist and a sociologist, find themselves working together, it is usual for the sociologist to take the role of "layperson" in the interaction. This gives the psychiatrist the power to control the content of the communication. For example, the psychiatrist will have the socially mandated power to determine whether a patient is to be diagnosed as "mentally ill". The social scientist may have a different view about who should be labelled "mentally ill". However, because of disciplinary imperialism, the clinical biomedical diagnosis will be given priority. Thus the psychiatrist has more transformative capacity ($power_1$), and the relationship between the psychiatrist and the social scientist is unequal and potentially oppressive ($power_2$). We can say that the psychiatrist's representation of reality trumps that of the sociologist, but this is only likely to result in conflict if their representations are different and if the sociologist refuses to accept their lower status relative to the psychiatrist. When researchers share the *same* representation, the situation is unlikely to trigger conflict because neither of the actors' representations of the object for research co-operation is challenged. This does not mean that the power mechanisms do not exist, but simply that they are latent tendencies – present, but unexpressed. Similarly, when different representations exist, but do not result in different ways of acting, then co-operation might also work smoothly. For example, perhaps a medical doctor thinks that a patient is simply a hypochondriac with no real illness, while a psychologist thinks that the patient has a treatable psychological illness, yet they both agree that there is no need to prescribe medication.

However, it is rare that different representations lead to the same action and therefore conflict frequently ensues. Often the conflict that arises is not merely between individuals, but also between cultures. For instance, a cultural clash is likely to occur in a team made up of two research communities – one invested in social constructivism and one invested in positivism – since these two groups have incompatible world views. An advantage of a critical realist approach is that such a conflict does not occur since its layered version of (intransitive) ontology creates a unique space for each discipline, whilst acknowledging that different methods and methodologies will be appropriate for each layer (ontological realism). However, because critical realism acknowledges that ontology is distinct from epistemology, it also creates a space for the social component of knowledge (the transitive dimension). There is therefore a kind of epistemological pragmatism at work, in which researchers use the language best suited to their particular purpose (epistemological relativism) and this can lead to each discipline using significantly different vocabulary, concepts, and models to conceptualize a particular problem. Nevertheless, this does not mean that researchers cannot understand each other, although it may take time and effort. Neither do they necessarily need to fully understand a discipline to benefit from its findings. Thus interdisciplinarity involves division of labour. Efficiency suggests that in some cases one only needs to learn enough of the language of a different discipline to be able to make use of its findings. For example, a linguist who has no background in statistics can nevertheless make use of statistical insights provided by a quantitative sociologist. Similarly, a quantitative researcher who has no background in qualitative interviewing can nevertheless make use of qualitative findings. If we do not ourselves have enough understanding to critically inspect a truth claim outside our discipline, it is necessary to trust independent reviewers. This is why trustworthy peer-reviewed publications – which have long been an important part of our academic arena – are vital in interdisciplinary settings.

Power behind representation

Following Fairclough's distinction, we can also analyse representation in terms of the power behind it. As indicated by the model of four-planar social being that was introduced in Chapter 4 (and connected to the WHO/ICF schema in Figure 11.1), power *behind* representation corresponds to the level of social structure, whereas power *in* representation corresponds to the level of interaction between agents.

In considering power behind representation, first, there are *structural* conditions that influence the constitution of the institutional practices of the researchers involved in the co-operation. At this level we can differentiate different spheres of power such as, for example, power in the economic system, the state, and interested organizations. For instance, after the discovery of the bacterial cause of peptic ulcer, the discoverers faced enormous resistance to their findings due in no small part to the structural power of commercial drug companies who had a vested interest in the existing regime of treatment. Furthermore, although the way that a powerful agent can impose a jargon upon other professionals is an example of power *in* social representations, this is nevertheless a result of structural conditions, i.e. power *behind* social representation. This type of power is anchored in such things as legislation, professional status, gender, and distribution of economic resources.

Second, power behind representations can be provided at the *institutional* level. The question here is how the practices, including enduring and internalized organizational forms, norms, and social relations, are constituted. An important part of power at this level is neutralization and the generation of common sense (Fairclough, 2001: 76ff). *Neutralization* is a technique that allows the dominant, ideological representation to be assumed to be the *only* legitimate way of interpreting and understanding reality (TINA, i.e. There Is No Alternative). It insinuates that the favoured representation is simply common sense. In the case of peptic ulcer, there were several decades where the "common sense" explanation (representation) of the peptic ulcer was that it was due to stress and diet-ruled – this prevented alternative hypotheses from being taken seriously. Another example is that it is "common sense" that only randomized controlled trial studies can be used in evidence-based medicine.

In this chapter, we have explored the ways in which power *in* representation and power *behind* representation result in fertile ground for disciplinary imperialism. In so doing we have underscored a key point of our book, which is that a common metatheoretical understanding, based on the critical realist approach to science, potentially avoids these problems. It allows scientists whose subject matter is situated in non-empirical reality to take their place as equals at the table alongside those scientists whose subject matter is empirical.

14

INTERDISCIPLINARITY IN ACTION

Explaining the epidemiology of HIV

What follows in this chapter is an illustration of the use of the DREI(C) in interdisciplinarity research in a context of HIV education. The research objective was to use the currently available literature on HIV to give an interdisciplinary understanding of the HIV situation in southern Africa. The goal was to use this interdisciplinary understanding to devise ameliorative educational interventions. One of the key characteristics of the southern African HIV pandemic which this research needed to explain, among other things, was that the region has much higher rates of HIV than anywhere else in the world (UNAIDS, 2015).

When this research was first embarked upon, the generally accepted theory for the high rates of HIV in southern Africa was that patriarchal local cultures encouraged a lack of women-respecting sexual restraint. This led to multiple concurrent partnerships and left women powerless to negotiate safe sexual practices or to avoid sexual violence, which in turn increased the incidence of HIV (Gupta, 2000; Koenig and Moore, 2000; Kaye, 2004; Halperin and Epstein, 2004). Traditional culture, specifically southern African black culture, was assumed to be a cofactor of the disease (Sovran, 2013). For the purposes of this paper, we will call this theory the African Culture Theory. For example, Leclerc-Madlala, Simbayi, and Cloete (2009: 16) state:

> Even though polygyny in contemporary South Africa is not the only norm prescribing husband–wife relations, the cultural heritage of polygyny continues to legitimise sex with multiple and concurrent partners and presents a challenge to HIV prevention. In southern Africa, including South Africa, sex with multiple and concurrent partners in the context of poor and inconsistent male condom usage has been identified as the key behavioural driver of HIV.

138 Applied interdisciplinary research

Using the RRREI(C)

Initially, there was no reason to disagree with the African Culture Theory and therefore it was assumed that the appropriate critical realist model of science was the RRREI(C), designed for applied science, in which adequate theory is already available. As a preliminary exercise, a multidisciplinary literature review was carried out. The empirical details and the various disciplinary theories explaining these details were summarized using Bhaskar's laminated model of reality, described in Chapter 6 (Price, 2010, 2014a). An outline of the findings is provided in Figure 14.1. Note that this information was presented in an interdisciplinary way in terms of the transdisciplinary African Culture Theory, and therefore focused on gender issues. This represented the first of the three steps in the RRREI(C), namely:

resolution of the high levels of HIV rates in southern Africa – the complex event or phenomenon – into its components, involving a conjunctive multiplicity of causes;
abductive redescription or recontextualization (into the southern African context) of these components in an explanatorily significant way; and
retrodiction of these component causes to antecedently existing events or states of affairs.

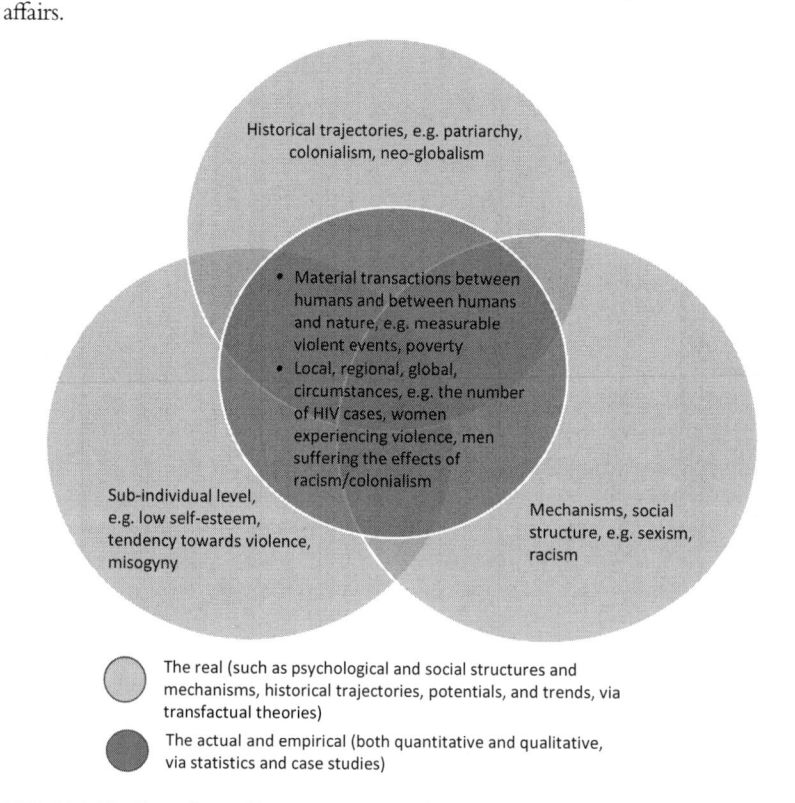

FIGURE 14.1 Findings from literature review theorizing the HIV situation in southern Africa

The evidence was not fully explained by orthodox theory

Once the evidence was collected, it was expected that it would be explained in terms of the mainstream African Culture Theory, describing the antecedent state of affairs. This would lead to suggestions for educational interventions. However, there was evidence that did not fit the African Culture Theory. As we made clear in Chapter 7, normal science proceeds in such a way as to test a generally accepted theory, that is, to confirm it, perhaps in a new context (this context was one of educational interventions). However, anomalies always exist in normal science and revolutionary science occurs when a new concept or a new theory is devised that avoids the anomalies. In this case, the normal science of the day was challenged by the following anomalies (Price, 2010):

- Traditional polygynous families, associated with gender inequality and examples of multiple concurrent partnerships, have some of the lowest rates of HIV prevalence in southern Africa (De Walque, 2006; Reniers and Watkins, 2010; Reniers and Tfaily, 2012).
- South African men with traditional patriarchal values have lower rates of HIV than men with modern patriarchal values (Kaufman et al., 2008).
- There are low rates of HIV in some societies with worse gender inequality and gender-based violence than found in southern Africa. For example, South Africans report less gender-based violence than people from Bangladesh, who have a much lower incidence of HIV (UNAIDS, 2007; Krug et al., 2002).
- Measures of sexual promiscuity, such as the sociosexual orientation index (Wellings et al., 2006; Schmitt, 2005), reveal that Western countries with low incidence of HIV are much more promiscuous than developing countries such as South Africa that have high incidence.

Essentially, certain epidemiological patterns of HIV infection challenge the African Culture Theory. Furthermore, some argue that the preoccupation with promiscuity in exotic groups – a fixation on the "sexual life of the natives" – is based on racist assumptions (Sovran, 2013). However, if African Culture is not responsible for the high rates of infection, then what is? To answer this question, it was necessary to use Bhaskar's DREI(C) model of pure science which contains the logic of retroduction, or the logic of theory building, where we develop theory that outlines the circumstances that must have existed to result in the situation that we are trying to explain.

Using the DREI(C): retroduction and elimination

The retroduction aspect of the DREI(C) is a creative process in which the researcher arrives at something new, perhaps even surprising, to better account for the empirical evidence. It usually entails the use of analogy and new vocabulary, or old vocabulary put to new uses. In this case, the key creative moment leading to the new theory was that the cultures associated with higher levels of HIV than the global average – southern African culture, intravenous drug user culture, and homosexual culture – were significantly similar in ways that potentially explained their increased susceptibility to HIV. However, because there was no usual way to describe the similarity among these groups, since on the surface they were significantly unlike each other, it was necessary to put old vocabulary to a new use. In this case, the old word to be put to a new use was "carnivalesque". The researcher therefore devised a theory around the idea that these cultures were similar and that these similarities could be summarized by describing them as cultures that reflect elements of the carnivalesque. The word was first used by Bakhtin and Kristeva (in Bové, 2006) to refer to theatrical challenges to the status quo. In this research, however, the definition is broadened to include a much wider variety of challenges than only the theatrical. However, the definition retains that aspect of "carnivalesque" that evokes behaviours that are simultaneously celebratory and/or pleasurable and challenging of the status quo. For example, gay culture, in certain of its manifestations, and as its name suggests, reflects the carnivalesque. Many southern Africans bravely challenge the globalizing, diversity-reducing *Gesellschaft* of neo-colonialism by insisting on maintaining the diversity of their culture. In this way, they embody the (far from frivolous) political aspect of the carnivalesque; perhaps think here of two popular South African leaders Nelson Mandela and Jacob Zuma. Both have directly challenged the Western norms of the behaviour of a head of state (consider Mandela's informal shirts and Zuma's polygynous lifestyle). Similarly, youth cultures associated with intravenous drug use, who also often challenge the norms of Western society, fit the carnivalesque description.

When deciding whether to use the word "carnivalesque", the following words were also considered: unconventional, festive, decorated, jubilant, celebratory, rogue, bohemian, bacchanalian, transgressive, subversive, couldn't-care-less, and nonconformist. However, these words were rejected because none captured both the elements of pleasure and resistance that exist in "carnivalesque". The risk of using the word carnivalesque is that it might seem to trivialize a powerful challenge to oppression. However, hopefully this risk was outweighed by the flip-side which is that the word carnivalesque does not suggest malicious disrespect for society. It may be true that the members of carnivalesque cultures embody a lack of respect for imposed rules, but their rebellion often tells a true story about the inequalities that they face, and therefore, whether they realize this or not, their actions are a significant political statement.

The Carnivalesque Theory

To explain the empirical evidence, it was argued that there is a healthy tendency for oppressed people to challenge and reject the rules of their oppressors. However, to rebel is risky. Furthermore, the rules of oppression are usually justified as something that is "good" for, or in the best interests of, the oppressed people: "The ideological complex thus represents the social order as simultaneously serving the interests of the dominant and the subordinate" (Hodge and Kress in Price,

2007: 157). In Chapter 10, we mentioned the so-called mental disease of drapetomania, whereby it was assumed that slaves who rebelled by running away must be mentally ill because it placed them into a jeopardous situation. In people who find themselves in strongly oppressive situations, it seems that the need for emancipation and personal empowerment sometimes renders issues of immediate safety irrelevant, since arguably there is no point in being safe if one is not free to enjoy that safety. Often, the motivation to conform to "good-for-you" rules, namely longevity and a fulfilled life, is absent for many oppressed people, since these human rights are denied to them. For example, Tadele (2000) found that following safer sex rules was of relatively low concern to street youths in Dessie due to their preoccupation with survival in an adverse environment. Dempster (2003) reported that truck drivers in Durban, South Africa consider the risk of unsafe sex to be minor in comparison to the other hardships of, and risks to, their lives. Furthermore, people cannot demonstrate to themselves that they have some freedom and that they are not completely oppressed – something they are likely to want to do to allow themselves some dignity – by always choosing the socially accepted options, that is, the options that are "good-for-you". Sadly, one of the few places where the oppressed can express their freedom without risk of legal or social sanction is in their personal lives; and often the socially frowned-upon behaviours in this context are materially and physically bad for them, such as unsafe sex, alcohol, and smoking. Even more unfortunate is that treating others badly, such as a wife or a member of a different marginal group, can also demonstrate a person's personal power to themselves, but unlike smoking, drinking, and unsafe sex, it is not immediately detrimental to the perpetrator, which perhaps(?) makes it all the more attractive. Ironically, transgressive behaviours that are self-destructive and destructive of others play into the hands of the oppressors and do not challenge the status quo. If anything, they can be used as proof by the oppressors that the oppressed are lesser human beings and therefore deserve to be low in the pecking order. This is analogous to Derrida's concept of the autoimmune condition (in Borradori, 2013/2003: 121) where mechanisms that are supposed to protect the organism become directed against it.

The Carnivalesque Theory therefore explains why, among other things (Price, 2010):

- in cultures where the sexuality of the women is usually strictly controlled, the cultural disposition is primarily conformist (to a non-modern, non-Western, traditionalist norm), and the men are generally not oppressed, there is relatively low HIV infection (e.g. Lebanon and Bangladesh);
- in cultures where the cultural disposition tends to be less traditional but nevertheless still conformist (to a modern, Western norm), and the men are generally not oppressed, there is also relatively low HIV infection (e.g. the UK and the USA);
- in cultures where the men as well as women generally face discrimination (such as due to their class, race, or sexual orientation), and there are relatively high levels of non-conformist behaviour, there tends to be a high rate of HIV infection (e.g. in southern African culture, gay male culture, and crack-user culture).

Two options of non-conformity

To explain further, in society we have at least two paths of non-conformity, both of which are risky in different ways, and both of which, it can be argued, are common in oppression-challenging, carnivalesque cultures:

- In the first path, non-conformity is a direct challenge to the status quo. One of the most visible, and at times socially dangerous, ways of doing this is through clothing or through the refusal to "be quiet" – literally by making noise, both aesthetic (singing, music, carnivals, colour) and conflictual (riots and demonstrations). Thus, carnivalesque actions can be described as sometimes shocking, colourful, and vibrant; think of Ghandi wearing his loincloth to meet with British officials; a youth covering her body with tattoos and piercings; Mandela's shirts; Zuma's chanting and singing; and gay pride.
- In the second path, non-conformity takes a self-destructive, abusive path (what should be healthy rebellion becomes an autoimmune condition). People rebelliously indulge in unsafe sex, dangerous recreational drugs, or act out violently against intimate partners.

Both these paths are consequences of a real tendency, namely, the tendency to react against structural oppression. The African Culture Theory uses the existence of the second path as evidence that southern African culture is problematic, and implies a moral judgement against southern Africans themselves. By contrast, the Carnivalesque Theory sees the second path as an unfortunate but explainable – and not inevitable – situation that is evidence of the global, neo-colonial oppression faced by southern African people. The African Culture Theory suggests actions that encourage southern Africans to change their culture, to become conformist to Western culture, and thus to stop challenging the world's oppressive status quo. It therefore demonizes southern African culture, blames the victims (hides the role of neo-colonialist racism and sexism), and provides a neo-colonial impetus. The Carnivalesque Theory celebrates southern African culture (seeing it as not necessarily represented by the second path that exhibits oppressive, sexist, violent tendencies), highlights the role of neo-colonialist racism and sexism, and supports the impulse towards freedom. Issues of gender are not ignored by the Carnivalesque Theory, instead they are seen as an exacerbating symptom of a broader discrimination against southern African people and their culture.

The positive correlations between multiple concurrent partners and HIV infection

It is, nonetheless, reasonable to ask about the positive correlations between multiple concurrent partners/promiscuity, gender-based violence, and HIV infection in individuals in certain populations (e.g. Dunkle et al., 2004; Neaigus et al., 2013; Pines et al., 2016). However, critical realism needs more than a correlation to admit causation, because of the open-system context. The Carnivalesque Theory explains these correlations, as well as a great deal more of the empirical evidence, because it suggests that disregarding the social norms of both monogamy and safer sex is often a reaction to oppression. The Carnivalesque Theory does not deny the potential for risky behaviour and gender-based violence to involve increasing the risk of HIV, but it does suggests that these are exacerbating symptoms – rather than causal – of a deeper problem. This is the same as the point that we made in Chapter 4, which is that we can prefer Einstein's theory over Newton's theory because it explains more of the evidence. Therefore, we can prefer the Carnivalesque Theory over the African Culture Theory because it explains more of the evidence. This process, of choosing a theory that explains more of the evidence, is called judgemental rationality.

A clash of research assumptions

When the research was sent for review, the reviewers agreed that conventional explanations were inadequate to explain the epidemiological evidence of the HIV pandemic. They also admitted that, compared to conventional explanations, the Carnivalesque Theory provided a better explanation of the evidence for the patterns of HIV. Nevertheless, they disapproved of the research. Their reasons for their disapproval were:

- They criticized the researcher for making the mistake of suggesting "a grand theory" and that this theory could not account for the unavoidable exceptions.
- They argued that the theory was problematic because it had not been proven through statistical testing and that a large-scale quantitative argument had not yet been made.
- They argued that the theory exhibited inappropriate stereotyping or generalization.

Answering the criticisms

Both postmodern and empiricist perspectives are wary of transfactual theoretical claims (Chapter 3). However, as we have explained at length, transfactual theorizing is a valid way of determining knowledge; and exceptions do not necessarily invalidate such theories because of the open-system context. The irony of having to state the need to achieve transfactual theories to achieve true interdisciplinarity is that – and this is an example of the TINA compromise formation described in Chapter 7 – scientists cannot avoid using transfactual truths about transcendental objects in their work. Note that the accepted African Culture Theory is also a transfactual theory, which can be criticized as being a grand theory and unproven. However, because transfactual theorizing is not mentioned in descriptions of mainstream science, it is possible for commentators to strategically choose which theories to criticize as unscientific. In this case, mainstream commentators choose to criticize the

Carnivalesque Theory because it challenges the status quo, while turning a blind eye to the grand theory, unproven status of the African Culture Theory. Some interdisciplinary, transfactual theorists whose theories have attracted the criticism of being unscientific, most likely for the same reason (that they challenged society's status quo), include: Sigmund Freud (theory of psychoanalysis); Simone de Beauvoir (theory of the mechanism of the oppression of women); Charles Darwin (theory of evolution); and Karl Marx (theory of the capitalist oppression of workers). All of these powerful theories were interdisciplinary and all of their authors were multi-disciplinary in their interests. Nevertheless, all of these scientists had to face accusations against their academic/scientific reputations (Price, 2012: 4).

One way to destroy an argument is to demonstrate that the content of the argument, the basic claims of its knowledge, is incorrect. The other, more devastating way, is to demonstrate that the method by which the knowledge claim was derived, that is, its basic epistemology, is flawed. Much of the content of the theories of de Beauvoir, Freud, Marx, and Darwin was deeply uncomfortable for many people and therefore it was advantageous for their critics to put into question the very epistemology upon which the theories were based. The Carnivalesque Theory is similarly uncomfortable for many people as it challenges certain religious or feminist positions. Specifically, it challenges those who strategically use the African Culture Theory orthodoxy to achieve their (feminist or Christian) moral goals of insisting on monogamy, compliance to (religious) sexual "norms", and gender equality. There are arguably very good reasons to avoid polygyny, sexually promiscuity, or sexism. However, the Carnivalesque Theory suggests that the risk of contracting HIV need not be one of them. Similar to the way that Darwin's theory challenged the idea that humans are created in the image of God, or Copernicus' theory challenged the idea that humans are the centre of the universe, so this theory challenges many people's assumption that HIV is God's (or perhaps some other naturalistic) punishment of those who are polygynous, gay, or sexist. Underlying this is another assumption, namely of the inherent superiority of Western cultural norms. Note how the critics of the Carnivalesque Theory did not argue with the content of the paper, but with its epistemology. Note also that their criticisms of the theory were similar to the pessimistic denials of interdisciplinarity, which we discussed in Chapter 3.

The way to decide whether a theory is valid is by judgemental rationality; therefore, we can take the Carnivalesque Theory seriously because it explains more of the evidence than the African Culture Theory. Validity is not through statistical, empirical generalizations, but through the adequacy of the explanation. It would be difficult to devise experiments to test such a social theory; perhaps it would be impossible to do so because of ethical considerations. Furthermore, science is a collaborative affair and most scientists do not complete all the stages of science on their own. In this case, the researcher used empirical evidence gathered from many other scientific sources to come up with the theory. Empiricist science tends to focus on the early stages of science, namely the descriptive, empirical fact-finding stage. Retroductive stages, such as demonstrated in this research, come later, when a significant amount of empirical evidence has been collected.

We can counter the reviewers' criticism that the Carnivalesque Theory is stereotyping and generalizing, by taking the position of the feminist Warren (1990), namely that identifying certain characteristics with certain groups of people is in itself an innocuous exercise. It is the motive behind the generalization that is important. For example, if one's objective is to achieve gender equality, it is counter-productive to begin by claiming that men and women are the same. We can only provide women with equal access to work if we acknowledge their differences from men – for instance, they have different childcare responsibilities, due to both cultural and biological reasons. We can only have discussions about the relevant differences between men and women if we have a concept of a concrete universal women, ontologically populated by unique, concrete singular women (cf. Chapter 7). Some feminists may be offended by the suggestion that women need special consideration, such as childcare facilities, in order to be treated equally, since this could be interpreted as perpetuating the stereotype that women are not as efficient workers as men. However, to fail to define women and their needs would be to greatly reduce the agency of women to achieve equality, by denying them tailored support. In the same way, we regularly tailor the workplace to suit the biology of men, for example, the heights of doors or the circumference of the grips on tools are matched to average male sizes. It is only because men are unmarked as the "other" that we do not notice the tailoring that accompanies their apparently seamless existence in the world.

Interdisciplinarity challenges us and requires reflexivity

We can also use this example of interdisciplinary transfactual theorizing to illustrate three other aspects of interdisciplinarity, namely that: it challenges our actions; it requires reflexivity; and it challenges our institutions.

Interdisciplinarity challenges our actions

In Chapter 7, we explained that to criticize a pre-existing belief, as happened in this research, is also to criticize the actions derived from that belief and ultimately it leads to more appropriate actions given the objective at hand (in this case, to reduce HIV infections). The action suggested by the African Culture Theory is that we should try to change African culture, making it into the likeness, one assumes, of Western culture. If African culture is the problem, then Christian, Western culture is seemingly the solution. The educational message becomes a form of neo-colonialism; it suggests that there is something inherently inferior about African culture and thus it perpetuates the oppression that the Carnivalesque Theory suggests is the reason for the extent of the HIV problem in the first place.

By contrast, the actions suggested by the Carnivalesque Theory are to do with preventing the oppression of the African people and refusing neo-colonialism. The powerful *joie de vivre* of the carnivalesque, which refuses to be oppressed, is exactly the aspect of this culture that gives its people hope and it is the energy of the carnivalesque that will hold them in good stead as they fight for their dignity and refuse to be oppressed. The challenge is how to guide this energy towards life-affirming rather than self-destructive activities, such as protected rather than unprotected sex. Questions of sexism are certainly not disallowed by this approach, but feminists should not use the threat of HIV to persuade men to be non-sexist or non-violent. Neither should Christians and those with a neo-liberal agenda use threats of HIV to achieve their objective of converting people to a Western, Christian lifestyle. Instead they should use the stronger, more honest argument for equality, namely that there is an ethical need for men to respect other human beings. How much more satisfying for a man to say "I do not rape women because I care about them" rather than "I do not rape women because I am afraid of HIV"? Or "I am faithful to my wife because I love her" rather than "I am faithful to my wife because I am afraid of HIV"?

Interdisciplinarity requires reflexivity

In Chapter 7, we explained that self-conscious reflexivity results in us taking responsibility for our actions and avoiding theory–practice contradictions. However, in order to do this, it is necessary to be honest with ourselves about the reasons for our activities. The researcher in this case study was – and still is, but in a different way – a strong feminist who was nevertheless conditioned/shaped by the mainstream orthodox discourse around HIV. As evidence emerged that challenged the mainstream orthodoxy, the researcher became increasingly uncomfortable. Researchers need to be honest with themselves about the true motives for their work. In this case, if the motive had simply been to reduce HIV, then it should have been easy to take the information that traditional polygamists have lower rates of HIV infection and advocate traditional (fidelity-based) polygyny as an HIV prophylaxis, along with (fidelity-based) monogamy. Of course, it was not that simple; and what this anomaly revealed was that feminists (and Christians and other advocates of monogamy) are strategically using the African Culture Theory to support a hidden agenda. Specifically, it is useful for them to hide their real message (which for different reasons might be poorly received) behind a message of HIV prevention. Acknowledging this does not stop them from continuing to advocate their feminist or Christian message. It merely means that they ought to be more honest about it. However, the point here is that the researcher had to be self-reflexive in order to fully embrace the truth of the situation.

Interdisciplinarity challenges institutions

Another question, however, is why it has taken so long for the African Culture Theory to be replaced by a more adequate theory, since evidence of the anomalies has been available in the literature for some time. As Halperin and Epstein (2004: 4) noted, since exposure to greater numbers of sexual partners over a lifetime constitutes an obvious source of vulnerability to HIV, the African Culture Theory is not illogical, but nevertheless it is "teeming with assumptions and ultimately incorrect". In Chapter 7, we discussed how certain sets of beliefs function in such a way as to uphold particular institutions. The false belief that the sun moved around the earth was held in place because it justified the Church's position at the top of the hierarchy of society. Similarly, the African Culture Theory is held in place because it justifies the activities of a number of institutions with hidden agendas (often Christian or feminist), such as nongovernmental organizations, faith-based organizations, and funding organizations. It also justifies structural racism because it seems to suggest the superiority of Western (white) cultural norms.

Conclusion

Because antinomy is the current hegemonic approach to interdisciplinarity, coherent alternatives may seem suspicious. Presently, it is possibly risky to one's career as a practising scientist to carry out true interdisciplinarity, wherein the key logic is retroduction. This is because, if a theory is put forward that challenges the status quo, the absence of the concept of retroduction (which allows us to develop theory) in the accepted scientific canon allows such a theory to be deemed unscientific. This means that those with power can strategically choose which theories to accept and which to reject. To accept a theory, they simply need to turn a blind eye to its nature as a transfactual. In this case, the African Culture Theory is as much a transfactual as the Carnivalesque Theory, but it is not critiqued as such because it serves a (questionable) purpose. By admitting a common metatheoretical perspective that includes retroduction, we can move beyond epistemological mud-slinging between disciplines and focus on discussions about the content of our theories and whether they adequately consider all the available empirical evidence.

15

CONCLUDING CONSIDERATIONS

Critical realism is applicable to real-life issues and problems, and it results in trustworthy, reliable science. Since most of the reason for carrying out science is to make practical changes in the world, the core of critical realism is applied critical realism. Additionally, since the open system of the world is ontologically layered, plural, and inherently multimechanismed, any science that attempts to understand it must necessarily be interdisciplinary, and therefore we can make the further claim that applied critical realist science is simply another term for interdisciplinarity:

critical realism used to address real-life issues = applied critical realism = interdisciplinarity.

Metatheoretical unity

Throughout this book, one of our major claims is that a key component of interdisciplinarity is the need for metatheoretical unity, namely that scientists of all disciplines speak the same language of the dialectic of scientific discovery. This metatheory must support and encourage model-building, integration of knowledge, and so forth. Such activities are difficult to justify without considering ontological factors, since they beg the questions: Model ... of what? Integration of knowledge ... about what? The question we therefore set out in the beginning of this book was: What must the nature of reality be like for interdisciplinarity to be possible? Or more fully: What must the nature of reality be like for interdisciplinarity to be possible, and necessary, and such a strikingly pervasive (and talked about!) feature of our experience? However, we do not argue that all researchers must embrace a critical realist view of reality. The critical realist view as described here is simply our suggestion of a way to achieve a metatheory that addresses these important challenges. However, we are convinced that there is a "bottom line" – regarding views of reality – necessary for interdisciplinary research. This bottom line is the acceptance that there is a deep structure of reality and that we need metatheoretical unity (see e.g. Finkenthal, 2001; Nicolescu, 2006; Bel Habib, 1990; Bunge, 1993). We believe that, currently, critical realism provides the most plausible way to achieve this bottom line; and in turn, critical realism may be superseded by a better approach.

Interdisciplinary research needs disciplinarity

Although all the disciplines that are involved in interdisciplinary research must have a metatheory in common, nevertheless, there are many ways in which each discipline must be different or highly specific. A prerequisite for successful interdisciplinary research is that the members of the research team are at the edge of their discipline. Ontologically, however, despite their differences, they will share a common metatheory that includes the idea that reality has levels, structures, mechanisms, emergence, and so forth. Therefore, one member of the team may be trained in statistical methods and able to provide epidemiological information about a disease, and another may be trained in qualitative interview methods, able to provide cultural information about the transmission of the disease, but both should understand that their referents (people infected, culture) are components of the layered ontology of the bigger research question, which is what causes the disease. Epistemologically and methodologically, the research team must therefore be specific in terms of where their research is located in the overall research process and have an understanding of the structures and mechanisms that might contribute to answering the questions related to the phenomenon under investigation, i.e. the members of the research team must be skilled, well-informed researchers, able to apply research methods relevant to their context.

For instance, at this time in 2016, our research of the Zika virus is still in its early stages – we are still looking for corroborating, confirming instances that demonstrate that the Zika virus is truly associated with microcephaly – and this requires laboratory work and includes inductive and deductive reasoning. However, once this association is well-corroborated, we will then want to move on to retroduction to possible explanatory causes. We will want to know exactly how the Zika virus causes microcephaly and what has caused its sudden increase in activity. Furthermore, in order to make successful interventions, we will need to know how the disease is transmitted. If, as seems to be the case, Zika can be transmitted via sexual intercourse, then addressing the epidemic will also require that we have in-depth knowledge about the values in the affected society regarding the use of condoms; for instance, perhaps there are religious values preventing people from using this kind of protection. This illustrates the need for an interdisciplinary approach to the "Zika problem", including a number of different disciplines such as biomedicine and anthropology.

Typically, rivals of critical realist versions of science describe just one moment of the research process (such as classical empiricism or Popper's falsificationism) but critical realism describes the entire research cycle and thus includes not just deduction and induction but retroduction, and indeed the entire transdictive complex. The Zika example highlights the need to include a number of ontological levels in the analysis, i.e. reality is a necessarily laminated system. At this moment in time, when we know so much about empirical reality, it is not surprising that the need for critical realism has become urgent as scientists intuitively realize that they are being limited by their narrow approach to epistemology.

Some problems associated with the absence of a depth ontology

In this book, we use the example of the International Classification of Functioning, Disability and Health (ICF) to demonstrate how the lack of a depth ontology can limit researchers' interdisciplinary engagement with the world. We argue that the ICF conceptual framework should be expanded to include both ontological and epistemological dimensions. By doing this, researchers will be able to use the ICF to engage in transfactual theorizing about the interdisciplinary causal explanations for health phenomena. Currently, these theories are the subject of antinomy in mainstream science and are avoided in the ICF because Humean-based philosophy denies the reality of the "something" that these theories are about. Therefore, while theories abound, there is no acknowledgement of their basis in a depth ontology; this basis would give them greater "social standing" – we would be allowed to take them more seriously. At the moment, they can only be taken seriously if respected experts choose to give them credibility by "looking the other way" so to speak, that is, by ignoring the Humean-based accusation that theories lack substance. Similarly, professionals working in the field of mental disability have categorized mental health disorders in the Diagnostic and Statistical Manual of Mental Disorders (DSM-5), but their Humean-based philosophy denies the reality of the "something" that their categories are about and therefore they have had to resort to calling their categories "fictive placeholders". By contrast, critical realists are realists about both theories (i.e. dispositions) and categories.

The concrete universal and the concrete singular

Nevertheless, critical realists do not naively think that there is a one-to-one correspondence between universal (transfactual) categories and theories, and empirical reality. Instead, they accept that a category or a theory can be either universal or expressed actually/empirically, but not both. This is because of the open system of the world in which regular constant conjunctions of events are practically impossible. In terms of categories, this means that whenever we are working with a category, say, bipolar disorder, we need to know its concrete universal characteristics but when dealing with a particular bipolar patient, we must acknowledge that the disease will be uniquely expressed depending on mediations such as the person's (concrete singular) other health issues, their psychological disposition, their social support network, etc. In terms of theories (and dispositions), it means that a theory may be true but not expressed due to factors that prevent its expression, or it may only be partially expressed. For example, the theory that racism is present in a culture may be true, but there may be no empirical expressions of racism due to the mediating factor of careful policing of behaviour. A person may have a genetic disposition towards alcoholism, but this disposition may never be expressed due to mediating environmental or social factors (the person may belong to a religion that prohibits alcohol).

Major difference between critical realism and rival accounts of science

We can summarize the major difference between critical realist accounts of science, and rival accounts, as being that critical realism prioritizes ontology whereas other approaches prioritize epistemology. Therefore, the main aim of critical realist researchers is exploratory probing of reality. They want to identify or discover, test the boundaries of, or uncover the structures of, impediments to, and causes of a phenomenon and to demonstrate how these coalesce, occur over time, and interact. They are therefore interested in transfactual or theoretical generalizing – arriving at transfactual concrete universals or theories – rather than empirical generalizations. This is contrary to the objectives of positivists and constructivists who prioritize epistemology and therefore want to prove/disprove/justify propositions and theories and who can only conceive of universals as empirical generalizations. This significantly limits what they can say about the world (for social constructionists it suggests that they can say nothing true about the world) and reduces the part of the world that most researchers feel comfortable to talk about to the empirical part. This denial of the ontological level of real structures and mechanisms, known as actualism, leads to the dual mistakes of reductionism and atomism.

Reductionism and atomism

Reductionism is the artificial reduction of a complex nexus of causal mechanisms, to a single underlying type of mechanism. Typically, in the health and wellbeing sciences, reductionism is often expressed as the reduction of causality to a biophysical cause. For example, it is the reduction of the cause of Attention Deficit Hyperactivity Disorder (ADHD) to a chemical imbalance in the brain (monodisciplinarity).

Atomism is the acknowledgement that there are several components to an issue, and while it is acknowledged that these interact, it is also said there is no overall theory that links them all together in a truly interdisciplinary way (multidisciplinarity). If we return to the example of ADHD, atomism acknowledges that ADHD includes genetic, social, economic, and biophysical issues. However, to achieve interdisciplinarity, it is necessary to creatively arrive at a theory of ADHD that provides a model (of the structures and mechanisms) that demonstrates how all of the issues are significantly related. One such theory (which we use here for illustrative purposes and do not necessarily advocate) is that ADHD is one mode of psychological being amongst many present in humanity, and that the mechanism which results in its presence in human populations is evolution, since ADHD bestows advantages and disadvantages on individuals and society (Bhandari and Khanal, 2016; Jaarsma and Welin, 2012). This theory combines all the components of ADHD – genetic, social, economic, and behavioural – to provide an interdisciplinary explanation for it. Such a theory needs to be systematically compared to competing theories to ascertain that it explains more of empirical reality than its rivals. For instance, a competing theory is that ADHD is simply a maladaptive brain anomaly (the mechanism here is random genetic mutation) but this does not explain the persistence and frequency of the condition in human populations.

Having introduced the idea of reductionism, we nevertheless need to explain that not all research that reduces the world into its components is necessarily reductionist. Perhaps we should qualify this idea by saying that critical realism critiques a priori reductionism. One version of a priori reductionism, sometimes called scientism – which has become increasingly popular as a result of our expanding knowledge about the genetic structures of human beings and the fast technological developments that have increased our ability to study the structure and functioning of our brain – advocates the universal applicability of the methods used in natural sciences. For these reductionists, empirical science is the only worthwhile worldview. For instance, Wilson (1999) claims that we can reduce the study of the social and cultural world (e.g. social behaviour, art, and technology) to basic bio-chemistry (e.g. to understanding the neurological categories that might explain the social or creative experience). Another version of a priori reductionism is social constructionism. Here everything is reduced to a social construction. For instance, Butler (2011) claims that gender is merely a social construct, with no basis in biology. However, critical realists (such as Gunnarsson, 2013 and Griffiths, 2016) assume that gender has both socially constructed and biological components. In another example, a social constructionist researcher might a priori assume that electromagnetic hypersensitivity is a social construction, ruling out the role of biological and psychological mechanisms involved in the development of the condition. Both types of a priori reductionism – associated with scientism and social constructionism – in their different ways reflect the epistemic fallacy, which is the reduction of ontology to epistemology. Both imply that there is no need for interdisciplinarity. This disjunctive causality approach (the phenomenon is caused by this or that underlying principle) is highly problematic and must be replaced by an approach that considers the interplay between a multiplicity of mechanisms, while nevertheless assuming that their outcome is an empirical question. Eventually, the result could be that some mechanisms are more important than others, but this should be a conclusion reached as the result of the research, and should not be its point of a priori departure.

There is however a type of acceptable reduction that is related to the purpose of a particular study. Especially at the beginning of an investigation, it is often not possible, or even desirable, to fully grasp all the levels and therefore the researchers must purposively limit the scope of their activity. In such cases, the researchers are aware that they are leaving out mechanisms at other levels and that they will not know the importance of these missing factors in relation to the phenomenon they are investigating. Because they have deliberately omitted parts of the whole, they must be transparent about how this limits their contribution in their research conclusions. This kind of reduction is acceptable because it is a necessary division of labour and it is not reductionist in the final analysis because the findings from this kind of research will, one assumes, in the end contribute towards the larger interdisciplinary picture of the issue. Using the Zika virus example, scientists could not begin to research the role of culture in the virus's transmission until they knew that it was sexually transmitted. They therefore had to begin with a narrow focus on the biological transmission mechanisms of the virus.

Instead of reductionism, we advocate a laminated system that includes a multiplicity of different mechanisms at a multiplicity of different levels. But we also believe that it is important to encourage pluralism, or substantive theoretical tolerance, at any one level, so as to allow the rational choice of the best among competing theories. Each level of reality requires its own theories, concepts, and methods. However, the distinct levels and mechanisms cannot be understood as separate and disengaged from each other in the reality we are studying, with correspondingly separable outcomes. In other words, they do not exist in a "vacuum" at any one level. Processes at one level are influenced by processes at another level. It is absolutely essential that the team members learn from each other but at the same time they must not lose the focus of their own field of expertise, i.e. they must find the correct balance between a disciplinary and an interdisciplinary focus, as the mechanism at "their" level will be influenced and affected by the mechanisms at other levels.

The ontology of interdisciplinarity

In terms of the ontology of interdisciplinarity, the reason that we need interdisciplinarity is because, with the exception of experimentally closed-context systems (and perhaps a very few naturally occurring systems), there are always a multiplicity of causes and mechanisms required to explain an event or concrete phenomenon. However, to move from multimechanismicity to multidisciplinarity and interdisciplinarity, we must also discuss emergence. Take the example of the way that society is emergent from people. To understand society, we need to understand its emergent mechanisms and structures, which results in a whole new discipline, i.e. sociology, one with a different methodology and methods from the study of the characteristics of people as individuals. Of course, this has not stopped sociologists in the past from trying to reduce their understanding of society to their understanding of its individuals (methodological individualism).

This brings us to one of the epistemological considerations of interdisciplinarity, which is the need for the epistemological step of transdisciplinarity. Transdisciplinarity includes retroduction, which is the logical process by which we start from an observation and move to a theory that accounts for the observation, preferably by choosing the simplest and most likely explanation. In terms of understanding emergent society, we need transdisciplinarity to theorize the existence of interdisciplinary social mechanisms and structures that are not reducible to the people who daily reproduce them. In terms of the issue of ADHD discussed previously, researchers used transdisciplinarity to creatively apply the model of the mechanism of evolution to help them to provide an explanation for the phenomenon.

Crossdisciplinary understanding

However, transdisciplinarity is not the only epistemological consideration of interdisciplinarity. It also depends on crossdisciplinary understanding between the members of the research team. The possibility of such understanding depends on the principles of universal solidarity and axial rationality (Bhaskar, 2012/2002). Universal solidarity is the idea that, in principle, any human being can understand any other human being. Axial rationality is the idea that there is a basic way of understanding the world, or learning about it, that is common to all people and cultures and that is implicit in all science (and thus is a precondition for metatheoretical unity). This way of reasoning is based on the principle that there must be explanations for differences. This is the basic pattern of reasoning or learning in science. Axial rationality is demonstrated in every culture, from the most erudite theoretical science to the most commonplace activities, such as when people learn how to prepare food, drive cars, or use computers. This kind of learning depends on our capacity to recognize and correct mistakes and it is because scientists are capable of axial rationality that crossdisciplinary understanding is possible. Some claim that crossdisciplinary misunderstanding is simply unavoidable, that the disciplines are simply incommensurable, that researchers must necessarily talk past each other, and that they cannot learn from each other. We avoid such pessimism by emphasizing that interdisciplinary research needs a common metatheory, such as critical realism. Immanent critique – that is, critique that addresses contradictions within an intellectual position – is used by critical realists to engage in discussions and comparisons of theories or positions that appear incommensurable.

Furthermore, crossdisciplinary understanding can be hampered by the cognitive structures that dominate a particular discipline. So, for example, typically, economics does not include the language or cognitive structures that are conducive to understanding the social presuppositions of economic activity; neither does medicine usually consider the various aspects of the holistic "chain of care". Therefore, for an economist and a sociologist to embark on crossdisciplinary understanding, the economist is likely to need to be convinced via immanent critique that economics as it currently exists would benefit from an understanding of social presuppositions. Similarly, for a medical doctor and a holistic practitioner to embark on crossdisciplinary understanding, the medical practitioner may need to be convinced via immanent critique that medicine as it is currently practised could benefit from certain forms of holistic care. Of course, there may also be the necessity for immanent critique of sociology and holistic healing. The point here is simply that, in principle, an economist can understand a sociologist, and a medical doctor can understand a holistic practitioner, and vice versa.

Institutional support for crossdisciplinary understanding

We have in this book paid much attention to the integration of knowledge, i.e. in terms of integrating content, but we have also highlighted the process of integration, i.e. in terms of the interplay of individuals in order to learn from each other and thereby get a broader view of the issue under investigation (Klein, 1990). It seems likely that to support the occurrence of both epistemic integration (content integration) and crossdisciplinary understanding (process integration) it may be necessary to expand the education and training of the relevant researchers or professionals. This is especially relevant when we consider the difficulties faced by researchers from the "hard" natural sciences and the "soft" social sciences in understanding each other, as illustrated by the investigation of Canadian biomedical scientists' perception of the social sciences in health research discussed in Chapter 13 (Albert et al., 2008). There have been a number of efforts to broaden our approach in health and medical education. However, it seems that many educational systems still insist on "specialization" too early and too completely.

Furthermore, there is perhaps not enough funding and institutional support for ongoing professional learning through close collaboration with other professionals, acquaintance with leading journals such as *Social Science & Medicine*, attendance of conferences and seminars outside one's major field, etc. Although this is a time and resource-consuming process, the importance of this type of crossdisciplinary understanding cannot be underestimated. As Hollingsworth and Hollingsworth (2000) conclude, "Organizations that have recurring major discoveries have tended to be those in which there is a high degree of interaction among scientists across diverse fields of science" (242). Such interaction "increases the tendency for creativity and for breakthroughs to occur" (243). Practical recommendations for achieving interdisciplinarity are ubiquitous, such as the recommendation that there should be defined career paths for interdisciplinary researchers and ring-fenced funding for interdisciplinary activities (as summarized in Table 12.1). These institutional and practical recommendations are all necessary, but nevertheless they will not be successful in achieving effective interdisciplinarity unless the condition of metatheoretical unity is also well-established.

We must therefore aim for a situation in which graduates feel comfortable to work with others from different disciplines. However, there is an inherent tension involved in interdisciplinary work, which is that, in order to follow the development of one's own subject or area of knowledge, one needs to interact with colleagues from the same field and to become specialized in that field. It is rare, perhaps impossible, for a person to have the mental capacity to be a specialist in all the disciplines. It is therefore likely that, even in ideal circumstances, there will be challenges in communicating with colleagues who lack a shared background.

However, the feelings of frustration and alienation – of not fitting in – can, we believe, be greatly reduced if all of one's colleagues share one's metatheoretical assumptions. Furthermore, such shared assumptions facilitate trust and equality amongst co-workers. This is because behind methodological imperialism – the idea that some methodologies are a lesser science – is the idea that only one methodology, usually empirical science, is true science. If it is assumed that some disciplines and their associated methodologies are epistemologically superior to others, then it is a small step to the assumption that practitioners of these methodologies deserve greater respect, leading to unequal social status among team members, and ultimately undermining true interdisciplinary co-operation.

Georges Gusdorf (in Klein, 1990: 19) argued that, "The need for interdisciplinarity has been reflected in epistemological writings ever since the origins of Western science". While this is true, nevertheless little has been written about interdisciplinarity from an in-depth ontological perspective. In this book, we have tried to overcome this shortcoming. We have done this by using critical realism to develop a metatheoretically sophisticated interdisciplinarity. Our aim is to help researchers to design sophisticated research procedures, to integrate the knowledge gained from the various individual disciplines, and to understand and apply knowledge in a more holistic way, thereby avoiding unilinear reductionism, additive atomism, and naïve eclecticism. We are convinced that global challenges in the field of health and wellbeing – as well as in the fields of global warming, terrorism, racism, and war – cry out for interdisciplinarity. By adopting a critical realist perspective that includes a laminated and emergent ontology and that facilitates metatheoretical unity, ameliorative interventions will be more successful than they are today.

REFERENCES

Albert, M., Laberge, S., Hodges, B. D., Regehr, G. and Lingard, L. (2008) Biomedical scientists' perception of the social sciences in health research. *Social Science and Medicine*, 66(12): 2520–2531.

American Psychiatric Association (1994) *Diagnostic and Statistical Manual of Mental Disorders (DSM)*. Washington, DC: American Psychiatric Association.

American Psychiatric Association (2013) *Diagnostic and Statistical Manual of Mental Disorders (DSM-5®)*. Arlington, VA: American Psychiatric Publications.

Archer, M. (2010) Morphogenesis versus structuration: on combining structure and action. *British Journal of Sociology*, 61(S1) (Re-print in 60th Birthday Issue of *British Journal of Sociology*): 225–252.

Archer, M. (2013) *Social Origins of Educational Systems*. London and New York: Routledge.

Archer, M. and Vaughan, M. (1971) *Social Conflict and Educational Change in England and France: 1789–1848*. Cambridge: Cambridge University Press.

Aschner, P., Aguilar-Salinas, C., Aguirre, L., Franco, L., Gagliardino, J. J., de Lapertosa, S. G. and Vinocour, M. (2014) Diabetes in South and Central America: an update. *Diabetes Research and Clinical Practice*, 103(2): 238–243.

Balkin, J. M. (1996) Interdisciplinarity as colonization. *Washington and Lee Law Review*, 53(3): 949–970.

Bammer, G. (2015) Interdisciplinarity: less vague please. *Nature*, 526(7574): 506.

Becher, T. and Trowler, P. (2001) *Academic Tribes and Territories: Intellectual Enquiry and the Culture of Disciplines*. Buckingham: SRHE and Open University Press.

Beecher, H. K. (1955) The powerful placebo. *JAMA – Journal of the American Medical Association*, 159(17): 1602–1606.

Bel Habib, H. (1990) *Towards a Paradigmatic Approach to Interdisciplinarity in the Behavioural and Medical Sciences*. Research Report 90:10, University of Karlstad, Sweden.

Benedetti, F., Lanotte, M., Lopiano, L. and Colloca, L. (2007) When words are painful: unraveling the mechanisms of the nocebo effect. *Neuroscience*, 147(2): 260–271.

Benedetti, F., Mayberg, H., Wager, T., Stohler, C. and Zubieta, J. (2005) Neurological mechanisms of the placebo effect. *The Journal of Neuroscience*, 25(45): 10390–10402.

Bermúdez, J. L. (2014) *Cognitive Science: An Introduction to the Science of the Mind*. Cambridge: Cambridge University Press.

Bernstein, B. (1971) *Class, Codes and Control: Theoretical Studies Towards a Sociology of Language*. London: Routledge and Kegan Paul.

Bhandari, P. and Khanal, P. (2016) Pride in autistic diversity: against treatment or for inclusion? *The Lancet*, 388(10059): 2477.

Bhaskar, R. (2000) *From East to West: Odyssey of a Soul*. London: Routledge.

Bhaskar, R. (2008a/1975) *A Realist Theory of Science*. London: Routledge.

Bhaskar, R. (2008b/1993) *Dialectic: The Pulse of Freedom*. London: Routledge.

Bhaskar, R. (2009/1986) *Scientific Realism and Human Emancipation*. London: Routledge.

Bhaskar, R. (2010) Contexts of interdisciplinarity. In R. Bhaskar, C. Frank, K. G. Høyer, P. Naess, and J. Parker (eds.), *Interdisciplinarity and Climate Change: Transforming Knowledge and Practice for Our Global Future*. London: Routledge, pp. 2–24.

Bhaskar, R. (2011/2002) *Reflections on MetaReality: Transcendence, Emancipation and Everyday Life*. London: Routledge.

Bhaskar, R. (2012/2002) *The Philosophy of MetaReality: Creativity, Love and Freedom*. London: Routledge.

Bhaskar, R. (2014/1979) *The Possibility of Naturalism: A Philosophical Critique of the Contemporary Human Sciences*. London: Routledge.

Bhaskar, R. (2016) *Enlightened Common Sense: The Philosophy of Critical Realism*. London: Routledge.

Bhaskar, R. and Danermark, B. (2006) Metatheory, interdisciplinarity and disability research: a critical realist perspective. *Scandinavian Journal of Disability Research*, 8(4): 278–297.

Bhaskar, R., Frank, C., Høyer, K. G., Naess, P. and Parker, J. (eds.) (2010) *Interdisciplinarity and Climate Change: Transforming Knowledge and Practice for Our Global Future*. New York: Routledge.

Bickenbach, J. E., Chatterji, S., Badley, E. M. and Ustun, T. B. (1999) Models of disablement, universalism and the International Classification of Impairments, Disabilities and Handicap. *Social Science and Medicine*, 48(9): 1173–1187.

Bogh, M. K., Schmedes, A. V., Philipsen, P. A., Thieden, E. and Wulf, H. C. (2010) Vitamin D production after UVB exposure depends on baseline vitamin D and total cholesterol but not on skin pigmentation. *Journal of Investigative Dermatology*, 130(2): 546–553.

Bordons, M., Morillo, F. and Gómez, I. (2004) Analysis of crossdisciplinary research through bibliometric tools. In H. F. Moed, W. Glänzel and U. Schmoch (eds.), *Handbook of Quantitative Science and Technology Research: The Use of Publication and Patent Statistics in Studies of S&T Systems*. Dordrecht: Kluwer, pp. 437–456.

Borradori, G. (2013/2003) *Philosophy in a Time of Terror: Dialogues with Jurgen Habermas and Jacques Derrida*. Chicago, IL: University of Chicago Press.

Bové, C. M. (2006) *Language and Politics in Julia Kristeva: Literature, Art, Therapy*. Albany: State University of New York Press.

Bowker, G. C. and Star, S. L. (2000) *Sorting Things Out: Classification and its Consequences*. Cambridge, MA: MIT Press.

Bradshaw, J. L. and Sheppard, D. M. (2000) The neurodevelopmental frontostriatal disorders: evolutionary adaptiveness and anomalous lateralization. *Brain and Language*, 73(2): 297–320.

Brancati, F. L., Kao, W. L., Folsom, A. R., Watson, R. L. and Szklo, M. (2000) Incident type 2 diabetes mellitus in African American and white adults: the Atherosclerosis Risk in Communities Study. *JAMA – Journal of the American Medical Association*, 283(17): 2253–2259.

Bratby, P. (2010) *Memorandum Submitted by Phillip Bratby: The Disclosure of Climate Data from the Climatic Research Unit at the University of East Anglia-Science and Technology Committee* (Memorandum No. CRU 17). London: House of Commons. Retrieved 19 May 2015 from http://www.publications.parliament.uk/pa/cm200910/cmselect/cmsctech/387b/387we18.htm

Brendel, D. H. (2003) Reductionism, eclecticism, and pragmatism in psychiatry: the dialectic of clinical explanation. *The Journal of Medicine and Philosophy*, 28(5–6): 563–580.

Brown, G. (2009) The ontological turn in education: the place of the learning environment. *Journal of Critical Realism*, 8(1): 5–34.

Bruyère, S., VanLooy, S. and Peterson, D. (2005) The International Classification of Functioning, Disability and Health (ICF): contemporary literature overview. *Rehabilitation Psychology*, 50(2): 113–121.

Bunge, M. (1993) *Causality and Modern Science*. New York: Dover Classics.

Burroughs, W. J. (2007) *Climate Change: A Multidisciplinary Approach*. Cambridge: Cambridge University Press.

Butler, J. (2011) *Gender Trouble: Feminism and the Subversion of Identity*. London: Routledge.

Chou, C. (1983) Splanchnic and overall cardiovascular hemodynamics during eating and digestion. *Federation Proceedings*, 42(6): 1658–1661.

Clark, S. G., Steen-Adams, M. M., Pfirman, S. and Wallace, R. L. (2011) Professional development of interdisciplinary environmental scholars. *Journal of Environmental Studies and Sciences*, 1(2): 99–113.

Cohrs, R. J., Martin, T., Ghahramani, P., Bidaut, L., Higgins, P. J. and Shahzad, A. (2015) Translational Medicine definition by the European Society for Translational Medicine. *New Horizons in Translational Medicine*, 2(3): 86–88.

Cole, S. W., Capitanio, J. P., Chun, K., Arevalo, J. M. G., Ma, J. and Cacioppo, J. T. (2015) Myeloid differentiation architecture of leukocyte transcriptome dynamics in perceived social isolation. *Proceedings of the National Academy of Sciences*, 112(49): 15142–15147.

Collier, A. (1989) *Scientific Realism and Socialist Thought*. Hemel Hempstead: Harvester Wheatsheaf.

Collins, R., Reith, C., Emberson, J., et al. (2016) Interpretation of the evidence for the efficacy and safety of statin therapy. *The Lancet*, 388(10059): 2532–2561.

Connolly, V., Unwin, N., Sherriff, P., Bilous, R. and Kelly, W. (2000) Diabetes prevalence and socioeconomic status: a population based study showing increased prevalence of type 2 diabetes mellitus in deprived areas. *Journal of Epidemiology and Community Health*, 54(3): 173–177.

Crawford, C. C. and Salmon, C. (2004) The essence of evolutionary psychology. In C. Crawford and C. Salmon (eds.), *Evolutionary Psychology, Public and Personal Decisions*. Mahwah, NJ: Erlbaum, pp. 23–49.

Cyna, A. M., McAuliffe, G. L. and Andrew, M. I. (2004) Hypnosis for pain relief in labour and childbirth: a systematic review. *British Journal of Anaesthesia*, 93(4): 505–511.

Danermark, B. (2002) Interdisciplinary research and critical realism: the example of disability research. *Alethia*, 5(1): 56–64.

Danermark, B. (2005) Handikappforskning som tvärvetenskap. Möjligheter och utmaningar [Disability research as interdisciplinarity]. In M. Söder (ed.) *Forskning om funktionshinder. Problem, utmaningar, möjligheter* [Research about Disability. Problems, Challenges and Possibilities]. Lund: Studentlitteratur, pp. 63–84.

Danermark, B. (2009) Kritisk realism och tvärvetenskap [Critical realism and interdisciplinarity]. In M. Bengtsson, A. Daoud and D. Seldén (eds.), *En realistisk sociologi i praktiken. Nio texter om samhället* [A Realist Sociology in Practice. Nine Texts about Society]. Göteborg: Sociologiska institutionen, Göteborgs universitet, pp. 51–68.

Danermark, B., Ekström, M., Jakobsen, L. and Karlsson, J. (2002) *Explaining Society: Critical Realism in the Social Sciences*. London: Routledge.

De Walque, D. (2006) *Who Gets AIDS and How? The Determinants of HIV Infection and Sexual Behaviors in Burkina Faso, Cameroon, Ghana, Kenya, and Tanzania* (Vol. 3844). Washington, DC: World Bank Publications.

Delbeq, A. I., Van de Ven, A. H. and Gustafson, D. H. (1975) *Group Techniques for Program Planning: A Guide to Nominal Group and Delphi Processes*. Glencoe, IL: Scott.

Dempster, C. (2003) South African men resist condoms. *BBC News*, 14 November, sec. Africa. http://news.bbc.co.uk/2/hi/africa/3268567.stm.

Denford, S., Frost, J., Dieppe, P., Cooper, C. and Britten, N. (2014) Individualisation of drug treatments for patients with long-term conditions: a review of concepts. *BMJ open*, 4(3): e004172.

Derrida, J. (1998) *The Derrida Reader: Writing Performances* (Vol. 15). Lincoln: University of Nebraska Press.

Dini, P., Iqani, M. and Mansell, R. (2011) The (im)possibility of interdisciplinarity: lessons from constructing a theoretical framework for digital ecosystems. *Culture, Theory and Critique*, 52(1): 3–27.

Donnelly, L. (2016) Biggest annual rise in deaths for almost fifty years prompts warnings of crisis in elderly care. *The Telegraph*. 16 February. Retrieved from http://www.telegraph.co.uk/news/health/12158930/Biggest-annual-rise-in-deaths-for-almost-fifty-years-prompts-warnings-of-crisis-in-elderly-care.html

Dunkle, K. L., Jewkes, R. K., Brown, H. C., Gray, G. E., McIntryre, J. A. and Harlow, S. D. (2004) Gender-based violence, relationship power, and risk of HIV infection in women attending antenatal clinics in South Africa. *The Lancet*, 363(9419): 1415–1421.

Durkheim, E. (2005/1897) *Suicide*. London: Routledge.

Engel, G. (1977) The need for a new medical model: a challenge for biomedicine. *Science*, 196(4286): 129–136.

Engel, G. (1981) The clinical application of the biopsychosocial model. *Journal of Medicine and Philosophy*, 6(2): 101–123.

European Commission (2014) FET – living interdisciplinarity. Retrieved 22 April 2016 from https://ec.europa.eu/programmes/horizon2020/en/news/fet-living-interdisciplinarity

European Union Research Advisory Board (EURAB) (2004) *Interdisciplinarity in Research*. EURAB 04.009-FINAL, Cordis Focus no. 245, 17 May 2004.

Evera, S. V. (1997) *Guide to Methods for Students of Political Science*. Ithaca, NY: Cornell University Press.

Everett, H. (1956) *Theory of the Universal Wavefunction*. Thesis, Princeton University, NJ.

Fairclough, N. (2001) *Language and Power*. 2nd edition. London: Routledge.

Ferrières, J. (2004) The French paradox: lessons for other countries. *Heart*, 90(1): 107–111.

Festinger, L. and Carlsmith, J. M. (1959) Cognitive consequences of forced compliance. *Journal of Abnormal and Social Psychology*, 58(2): 203–210.

Finkenthal, M. (2001) *Interdisciplinarity: Toward the Definition of a Metadiscipline?* American University Studies, Series V, Philosophy. Vol. 187. New York: Peter Lang.

Finniss, D. G., Kaptchuk, T. J., Miller, F. and Benedetti, F. (2010) Biological, clinical, and ethical advances of placebo effects. *The Lancet*, 375(9715): 686–695.

Fish, S. (1989) Being interdisciplinary is so very hard to do. *Profession*, 89: 15–22. Rpt. in *Interdisciplinarity: Essays from the Literature* (W. H. Newell, ed.). New York: College Entrance Examination Board, pp. 239–249.

Flood, R. and Jackson, M. (1991) *Creative Problem Solving: Total Systems Intervention*. Chichester: Wiley.

Fordham, G. (2014) *HIV/AIDS and the Social Consequences of Untamed Biomedicine: Anthropological Complicities*. London: Routledge.

Freud, S. (1923) Two encyclopaedia articles: psycho-analysis and the libido theory. *S.E.*, 18: 233–259.

Frodeman, R. (2014) *Sustainable Knowledge. A Theory of Interdisciplinarity*. New York: Palgrave Macmillan.

Garthwaite, K. (2014) Fear of the brown envelope: exploring welfare reform with long-term sickness benefits recipients. *Social Policy and Administration*, 48(7): 782–798.

Genius, S. J. and Lipp, C. T. (2012) Electromagnetic hypersensitivity: fact or fiction? *Science of The Total Environment*, 414: 103–112.

Giddens, A. (1986) *The Constitution of Society: Outline of the Theory of Structuration*. Cambridge: Polity Press.

Gilgun, J. (2001) *Case-based research, analysis induction, and theory development: the future and the past*. Presented at the 31st Annual Theory Construction and Research Methodology Workshop, National Council on Family Relations, Rochester, NY.

Godlee, F. (2016) Statins: we need an independent review. *BMJ*, 354: i4992.

Goodley, D. (2010) *Disability Studies: An Interdisciplinary Introduction*. London: Sage.

Greenhalgh, T., Snow, R., Ryan, S., Rees, S. and Salisbury, H. (2015) Six 'biases' against patients and carers in evidence-based medicine. *BMC Medicine*, 13: 200.

Gribbin, J. R. (2004) *Deep Simplicity: Bringing Order to Chaos and Complexity*. New York: Random House.

Griffiths, D. A. (2016) Queer genes: realism, sexuality and science. *Journal of Critical Realism*, 15(5): 511–529.

Gunnarsson, L. (2013) *The Contradictions of Love: Towards a Feminist-realist Ontology of Sociosexuality*. London: Routledge.

Gupta, G. (2000) Gender, sexuality, and HIV/AIDS: the what, the why, and the how. *Policy Law Review*, 5(4): 86–93.

Halperin, D. T. and Epstein, H. (2004) Concurrent sexual partnerships help to explain Africa's high HIV prevalence: implications for prevention. *The Lancet*, 364(9428): 4–6.

Harding, S. G. (2004) *The Feminist Standpoint Theory Reader: Intellectual and Political Controversies*. New York: Psychology Press.

Hegel, G. W. F. (1998/1807) *Phenomenology of Spirit*. Delhi: Motilal Banarsidass.

Heinze, R. (2005) *Ethics of Literary Forms in Contemporary American Literature*. Münster: LIT Verlag.

Hensvold, A. H., Magnusson, P. K., Joshua, V., Hansson, M., Israelsson, L., Ferreira, R. and Askling, J. (2013) Environmental and genetic factors in the development of anticitrullinated protein antibodies (ACPAs) and ACPA-positive rheumatoid arthritis: an epidemiological investigation in twins. *Annals of the Rheumatic Diseases*, 74(2): 375–380.

Hepworth, J. (1999) *The Social Construction of Anorexia Nervosa*. London: Sage.

Higher Education Funding Council for England (2015) *Interdisciplinary Research using a Citation-based Approach: Report to the UK HE Funding Bodies and MRC*. London: Elsevier.

Hobbs, F. R., Banach, M., Mikhailidis, D. P., Malhotra, A. and Capewell, S. (2016) Is statin-modified reduction in lipids the most important preventive therapy for cardiovascular disease? A pro/con debate. *BMC Medicine*, 14: 4.

Holland, G. (2014) *Integrating Knowledge through Interdisciplinary Research. Problems of Theory and Practice*. London: Routledge.

Hollingsworth, R. and Hollingsworth, E. J. (2000) Major discoveries and biomedical research organizations: perspectives on interdisciplinarity, nurturing leadership, and integrated structure and cultures. In P. Weingart and N. Stehr (eds.), *Practising Interdisciplinarity*. Toronto: University of Toronto Press, pp. 215–244.

Holmberg, J. and Robèrt, K.-H. (2000) Backcasting from non-overlapping sustainability principles – a framework for strategic planning. *International Journal of Sustainable Development and World Ecology*, 7(4): 291–308.

Hope, K. W. and Waterman, H. A. (2003) Praiseworthy pragmatism? Validity and action research. *Journal of Advanced Nursing*, 44(2): 120–127.

Horenstein, R. B. and Shuldiner, A. R. (2004) Genetics of diabetes. *Reviews in Endocrine and Metabolic Disorders*, 5(1): 25–36.

Howe, K. R. (1988) Against the qualitative-quantitative incompatibility thesis or dogmas die hard. *Educational Researcher*, 17(8): 10–16.

Høyer, K. G. and Naess, P. (2008) Interdisciplinary, ecology and scientific theory: the case of sustainable urban development. *Journal of Critical Realism*, 7(2): 179–207.

Hu, F. B. (2011) Globalization of diabetes: the role of diet, lifestyle, and genes. *Diabetes Care*, 34(6): 1249–1257.

Hume, D. (1748) *An Enquiry Concerning Human Understanding. Of the Idea of Necessary Connexion*. Retrieved from http://www.bartleby.com/37/3/10.html

Hume, D. (1934/1740) *A Treatise of Human Nature, Vol. II*. London: J. M. Dent.

Hume, D. (2008/1779) *Dialogues Concerning Natural Religion*. Oxford: Oxford University Press.

Imrie, R. (2004) Demystifying disability: a review of the International Classification of Functioning, Disability and Health. *Sociology of Health and Illness*, 26(3): 287–305.

Jaarsma, P. and Welin, S. (2012) Autism as a natural human variation: reflections on the claims of the neurodiversity movement. *Health Care Analysis*, 20(1): 20–30.

Johansson, E. E., Risberg, G. and Hamberg, K. (2003) Is qualitative research scientific, or merely relevant? Research-interested primary care and hospital physicians' appraisal of abstracts. *Scandinavian Journal of Primary Health Care*, 21(1): 10–14.

Karhausen, L. R. (2000) Causation: the elusive grail of epidemiology. *Medicine, Health Care and Philosophy*, 3(1): 59–67.

Karlsen, S. and Nazroo, J. Y. (2002) Agency and structure: the impact of ethnic identity and racism on the health of ethnic minority people. *Sociology of Health and Illness*, 24(1): 1–20.

Kaufman, M., Shefer, T., Crawford, M., Leickness, C. and Kalichman, S. (2008) Gender attitudes, sexual power, HIV risk: a model for understanding HIV risk behavior of South African men. *AIDS Care*, 20(4): 434–441.

Kaunitz, H. (1977) The significance of dietary fat in arteriosclerosis. An outmoded theory? *MMW Munch Med Wochenschrift*, 119(16): 539–542.

Kaunitz, H. (1978) Cholesterol and repair processes in arteriosclerosis. *Lipids*, 13(5): 373–374.

Kaye, D. (2004) Gender inequality and domestic violence: implications for human immunodeficiency virus (HIV) prevention. *African Health Sciences*, 4(1): 67–70.

Kessel, F., Rosenfield, P. and Anderson, N. (eds.) (2008) *Interdisciplinary Research. Case Studies from Health and Social Science*. New York: Oxford University Press.

Kivimäki, M., Jokela, M., Nyberg, S. T., Singh-Manoux, A., Fransson, E. I., Alfredsson, L. and Clays, E. (2015) Long working hours and risk of coronary heart disease and stroke: a systematic review and meta-analysis of published and unpublished data for 603 838 individuals. *The Lancet*, 386(10005): 1739–1746.

Klein, J. T. (1990) *Interdisciplinarity. History, Theory, and Practice*. Detroit: Wayne State University Press.

Koenig, L. J. and Moore, J. (2000) Women, violence, and HIV: a critical evaluation with implications for HIV services. *Maternal Child Health*, 4(2): 103–109.

Krohn, W. (2010) Interdisciplinary cases and disciplinary knowledge. In R. Frodeman (ed.), *The Oxford Handbook of Interdisciplinarity*. Oxford: Oxford University Press, pp. 31–38.

Krug, E. G., Mercy, J. A., Dahlberg, L. L. and Zwi, A. B. (2002) The world report on violence and health. *The Lancet*, 360(9339), 1083–1088.

Kuhn, T. S. (2012/1962) *The Structure of Scientific Revolutions*. 50th Anniversary Edition. Chicago, IL: University of Chicago Press.

Kumari, M., Head, J. and Marmot, M. (2004) Prospective study of social and other risk factors for incidence of type 2 diabetes in the Whitehall II study. *Archives of Internal Medicine*, 164(17): 1873–1880.

Lather, P. (1991) *Getting Smart: Feminist Research and Pedagogy with/in the Postmodern*. New York: Psychology Press.

Leclerc-Madlala, S., Simbayi, L. C. and Cloete, A. (2009) The sociocultural aspects of HIV/AIDS in South Africa. In P. Rohleder, L. Swartz, S. Kalichman and L. Simbayi (eds.), *HIV/AIDS in South Africa 25 Years On*. New York: Springer, pp. 13–25.

Lehmkuhl, L. D. (1996) Nonparametric statistics: methods for analyzing data not meeting assumptions required for the application of parametric tests. *Journal of Prosthetists and Orthotists*, 8(3): 105–113.

Leighton, T. G. (2016) Are some people suffering as a result of increasing mass exposure of the public to ultrasound in air? *Proceedings of the Royal Society of London A*, 472(2185): 20150624.

Lincoln, Y. S. and Guba, E. G. (1985) *Naturalistic Inquiry: The Paradigm Revolution*. London: Sage.

Locke, J. (1979/1689) *An Essay Concerning Human Understanding* (P. H. Nidditch, ed.). Oxford: Clarendon Press.

Luhmann, N. (1997) Limits of steering. *Theory, Culture and Society*, 14(1): 37–39.

Mackey, J. L. (1995) Fractals or fish: does a space for interdisciplinarity exist? *Issues in Integrative Studies*, 13, 101–113.

McPherson, S. and Armstrong, D. (2006) Social determinants of diagnostic labels in depression. *Social Science and Medicine*, 62(1): 50–58.

Malhotra, A. (2013) Saturated fat is not the major issue. *BMJ*, 347: f6340.

Manyande, A. and Grabowska, C. (2009) Factors affecting the success of moxibustion in the management of a breech presentation as a preliminary treatment to external cephalic version. *Midwifery*, 25(6): 774–780.

Maturana, H. and Varela, F. J. (1987) *The Tree of Knowledge: The Biological Roots of Human Understanding*. Boston, MA: Shambhala.

Max-Neef, M. (2005) Foundations of transdisciplinarity. *Ecological Economics*, 53(1): 5–16.

Moody-Ayers, S. Y., Stewart, A. L., Covinsky, K. E. and Inouye, S. K. (2005) Prevalence and correlates of perceived societal racism in older African-American adults with type 2 diabetes mellitus. *Journal of the American Geriatrics Society*, 53(12): 2202–2208.

Moran, J. (2002) *Interdisciplinarity*. London: Routledge.

Morillo, F., Bordons, M. and Gómez, I. (2001) An approach to interdisciplinarity through bibliometric indicators. *Scientometrics*, 51(1): 203–222.

Mundasad, S. (2016, 16 February) Large 'jump in deaths' expert warns. *BBC News*. Retrieved from http://www.bbc.co.uk/news/uk-england-35589564

National Academy of Sciences (NAS) (2004) *Facilitating Interdisciplinary Research*. Committee on Science, Engineering, and Public Policy. Washington, DC: National Academies Press.

Neaigus, A., Jenness, S. M., Hagan, H., Murrill, C. S. and Wendel, T. (2013) Reciprocal sex partner concurrency and STDs among heterosexuals at high-risk of HIV infection. *Journal of Urban Health*, 90(5): 902–914.

Newell, W. (2001) A theory of interdisciplinary studies. *Issues in Integrative Studies*, 19: 1–25.

Nicolescu, B. (2006) Transdisciplinarity: past, present and future. In B. Haverkort and C. Reijntjes (eds.) *Moving Worldviews Reshaping Sciences, Policies and Practices for Endogenous*

Sustainable Development. COMPAS series on Worldviews and Sciences, No. 4. Leusden, The Netherlands: ETC/COMPAS, pp. 142–166.

Ninabahen, D. D., Xiang, L., Rehn, K. E. and Marshall, G. D. (2011) Stress and allergic diseases. *Immunology and Allergy Clinics of North America*, 31(1): 55–68.

Nowotny, H. (2004) The potential of transdisciplinarity. In H. Dunin-Woyseth and M. Nielsen (eds.), *Discussing Interdisciplinarity: Making Professions and the New Mode of Knowledge Production, the Nordic Reader*. Oslo, Norway: Oslo School of Architecture, pp. 10–19.

Nussbaum, A. M. (2013) On the origin of the specious: the evolution of the DSM–5. *PsycCRITIQUES*, 58(45): Article 2.

Odum, H. T. (1994) *Ecological and General Systems: An Introduction to Systems Ecology*. Revised Edition. Niwot, CO: University Press of Colorado.

Oreskes, N. (2007) The scientific consensus on climate change: how do we know we're not wrong? In J. DiMento and P. Doughman (eds.), *Climate Change: What It Means for Us, Our Children, and Our Grandchildren*. Cambridge, MA: MIT Press, pp. 65–99.

Organisation for Economic Co-operation and Development (2010) *Privatising State-owned Enterprises: An Overview of Policies and Practices in OECD Countries*. Paris: Organisation for Economic Co-operation and Development.

Palmer, C., Gothe, J., Mitchell, C., et al. (2007) Finding integration pathways: developing a transdisciplinary (TD) approach for the Upper Nepean Catchment. In A. L. Wilson, R. L. Dehaan, R. J. Watts, K. J. Page, K. H. Bowmer, and A. Curtis (eds.), *Australian Rivers: Making a Difference. Proceedings of the 5th Australian Stream Management Conference*. Charles Sturt University, Thurgoona, New South Wales, pp. 306–311.

Parker, J. (2010) Towards a dialectics of knowledge and care in the global system. In R. Bhaskar, C. Frank, K. G. Høyer, P. Næss, and J. Parker (eds.), *Interdisciplinarity and Climate Change: Transforming Knowledge and Practice for Our Global Future*. London: Routledge, pp. 205–226.

Pines, H. A., Wertheim, J. O., Liu, L., Garfein, R. S., Little, S. J. and Karris, M. Y. (2016) Concurrency and HIV transmission network characteristics among men who have sex with men with recent HIV infection. *AIDS*, 30(18): 2875–2883.

Pohl, C. (2005) Transdisciplinary collaboration in environmental research. *Futures*, 37(10): 1159–1178.

Polonsky, W. H., Fisher, L., Guzman, S., Villa-Caballero, L. and Edelman, S. V. (2005) Psychological insulin resistance in patients with type 2 diabetes: the scope of the problem. *Diabetes Care*, 28(10): 2543–2545.

Popper, K. (2014/1963) *Conjectures and Refutations: The Growth of Scientific Knowledge*. London: Routledge.

Popper, K. S. (2012/1945) *The Open Society and Its Enemies*. London: Routledge.

Price, L. (2007) *A Transdisciplinary Explanatory Critique of Environmental Education in Business and Industry*. PhD thesis. Rhodes University, Grahamstown.

Price, L. (2010) The carnivalesque factor in southern African HIV pandemic. *Exchange on HIV/AIDS, Sexuality and Gender*, 2: 3–7.

Price, L. (2012). Conceptualising interdisciplinarity: a precondition for a better world. Paper presented at the International Centre Critical Realism discussion series, April 24, 2012, Clarke Hall Education Department, Institute of Education. Retrieved from https://www.academia.edu/11200342/Conceptualising_interdisciplinarity_a_precondition_for_a_better_world

Price, L. (2014a) Critical realist versus mainstream interdisciplinarity. *Journal of Critical Realism*, 13(1): 52–76.

Price, L. (2014b) Hume's two causalities and social policy: moon rocks, transfactuality, and the UK's policy on school absenteeism. *Journal of Critical Realism*, 13(4): 385–398.

Price, L. (2016) Integrating knowledge through interdisciplinary research: problems of theory and practice. Dominic Holland. *Journal of Critical Realism*, 15(3): 320–322.

Priest, G., Beall, J. C. and Armour-Garb, B. (2004) *The Law of Non-contradiction: New Philosophical Essays*. Oxford: Oxford University Press.

Reniers, G. and Tfaily, R. (2012) Polygyny, partnership concurrency, and HIV transmission in sub-Saharan Africa. *Demography*, 49(3): 1075–1101.

Reniers, G. and Watkins, S. (2010) Polygyny and the spread of HIV in sub-Saharan Africa: a case of benign concurrency. *AIDS*, 24(2): 299–307.

Richter, D. (1999) Chronic mental illness and the limits of the biopsychosocial model. *Medicine, Health Care and Philosophy*, 2(1): 21–30.

Rittel, H. W. and Webber, M. M. (1973) Dilemmas in a general theory of planning. *Policy Sciences*, 4(2): 155–169.

Rodriguez, T. (2015) Beliefs can trigger asthma attacks. *Scientific American*. Retrieved 2 April 2016 from http://www.scientificamerican.com/article/beliefs-can-trigger-asthma-attacks/

Roland, M. and Guthrie, B. (2016) Quality and Outcomes Framework: what have we learnt? *British Medical Journal*, 354, i4060.

Röösli, M. (2008) Radiofrequency electromagnetic field exposure and non-specific symptoms of ill health: a systematic review. *Environmental Research*, 107(2): 277–287.

Rorty, R. (1982) *Consequences of Pragmatism: Essays, 1972–1980*. Minneapolis: University of Minnesota Press.

Rorty, R. (1989) *Contingency, Irony, and Solidarity*. Cambridge: Cambridge University Press.

Rosendahl, J., Zanella, M. A., Rist, S. and Weigelt, J. (2015) Scientists' situated knowledge: strong objectivity in transdisciplinarity. *Futures*, 65: 17–27.

Rowe, J. W. (2008) Introduction: approaching interdisciplinary research. In F. Kessel, P. L. Rosenfield, and N. B. Anderson (eds.), *Interdisciplinary Research. Case Studies from Health and Social Science*. New York: Oxford University Press, pp. 3–9.

Rubin, G. J., Hahn, G., Everitt, B. S., Cleare, A. J. and Wessely, S. (2006) Are some people sensitive to mobile phone signals? Within participants double blind randomised provocation study. *BMJ*, 332(7546): 886–891.

Ryan, A. M., Krinsky, S., Kontopantelis, E. and Doran, T. (2016) Long-term evidence for the effect of pay-for-performance in primary care on mortality in the UK: a population study. *Lancet*, 388(10041): 268–274.

Ryan, R. M. and Deci, E. L. (2008) A self-determination theory approach to psychotherapy: the motivational basis for effective change. *Canadian Psychology/Psychologie Canadienne*, 49(3): 186–193.

Sadler, J. Z. and Hulgus, Y. F. (1990) Knowing, valuing, acting: clues to revising the biopsychosocial model. *Comprehensive Psychiatry*, 31(3): 185–195.

Sadler, J. Z. and Hulgus, Y. F. (1992) Clinical problem solving and the biopsychosocial model. *American Journal of Psychiatry*, 149(10): 1315–1323.

Sample, I. (2010, September 29) Letters shed light on bitter rivalries behind discovery of DNA double helix. *The Guardian*. Retrieved from http://www.theguardian.com/science/2010/sep/29/letters-dna-double-helix-francis-crick

Sawa, R. J. (2005) Foundations of interdisciplinarity. *Medicine, Health Care and Philosophy*, 8(1): 53–61.

Sayer, A. (2000) *Realism and Social Science*. London: Sage.

Schmitt, D. (2005) Sociosexuality from Argentina to Zimbabwe: a 48-nation study of sex, culture, and strategies of human mating. *Behavioural and Brain Sciences*, 28(2): 247–311.

Scott-Samuel, A., Bambra, C., Collins, C., Hunter, D. J., McCartney, G. and Smith, K. (2014) The impact of Thatcherism on health and well-being in Britain. *International Journal of Health Services*, 44(1): 53–71.

Scriven, M. (1974) Exact role of value judgements in science. In K. Schaffner and R. S. Cohen (eds.), *Proceedings of the 1972 Biennial Meeting of the Philosophy of Science Association*. Dordrecht, Holland: Reidel Publishing, pp. 219–247.

Seldén, D. (2005) *Om det som är. Ontologins metodologiska relevans inom positivism, relativism och kritisk realism* [Concerning being. Ontology and its methodological relevance within positivism, relativism and critical realism]. Göteborgs Studies in Sociology, No. 24. Göteborg: Department of Sociology, Göteborgs universitet.

Sharfstein, S. (2005) Response to the presidential address: advocacy for our patients and our profession. *American Journal of Psychiatry*, 162(11): 2045–2047.

Siedlok, F. and Hibbert, P. (2014) The organization of interdisciplinary research: modes, drivers and barriers. *International Journal of Management Reviews*, 16(2): 194–210.

Skinningsrud, T. (2007) Realist social theorising and the emergence of state educational systems. In C. Lawson, J. S. Latsis and N. M. O. Martins (eds.), *Contributions to Social Ontology*. London: Routledge, pp. 252–272.

Sokolowski, R. (2008) *Phenomenology of the Human Person*. Cambridge: Cambridge University Press.

Sovran, S. (2013) Understanding culture and HIV/AIDS in sub-Saharan Africa. *Sahara Journal*, 10(1): 32–41.

Steinmetz, G. (1998) Critical realism and historical sociology. *Comparative Studies in Society and History*, 40(1): 170–186.

Stokols, D., Harvey, R., Gress, J., Fuqua, J. and Philips, K. (2005) In vivo studies of transdisciplinary scientific collaboration. *American Journal of Preventive Medicine*, 28(2 Suppl. 2): 202–213.

Stone, R. A., Maguire, M. G. and Quinn, G. E. (2000) Vision: reply: myopia and ambient night-time lighting. *Nature*, 404(6774): 144.

Strober, M. (2011) *Interdisciplinary Conversations: Challenging Habits of Thought*. Palo Alto, CA: Stanford University Press.

Stucki, G. and Grimby, G. (2007) Organizing human functioning and rehabilitation research into distinct scientific fields. Part I: developing a comprehensive structure from the cell to society. *Journal of Rehabilitation Medicine*, 39(4): 293–298.

Stucki, G., Reinhardt, J. D., Grimby, G. and Melvin, J. (2007) Developing "human functioning and rehabilitation research" from the comprehensive perspective. *Journal of Rehabilitation Medicine*, 39(9): 665–671.

Swedish Research Council (Vetenskapsrådet) (2005) *Tvärvetenskap – en analys*. Vetenskapsrådets rapportserie 10:2005. Stockholm: Vetenskapsrådet.

Tadele, G. (2000) *Bleak Prospects: Young Men, Sexuality and HIV/AIDS in an Ethiopian Town*. Leiden: African Studies Centre.

Tashakkori, A. and Teddlie, C. (1998) *Mixed Methodology. Combining Qualitative and Quantitative Approaches*. Applied Social Research Methods Series, vol. 46. Thousand Oaks, CA: Sage.

Taylor, M. C. (2010) *Crisis on Campus: A Bold Plan for Reforming Our Colleges and Universities*. New York: Alfred A. Knopf.

Tesh, S. N. (1988) *Hidden Arguments: Political Ideology and Disease Prevention Policy*. New Brunswick, NJ: Rutgers University Press.

Turner, B. S. (1990) The interdisciplinary curriculum: from social medicine to postmodernism. *Sociology of Health and Illness*, 12(1): 1–23.

UNAIDS (2007) Country factsheet. Retrieved from http://www.unaids.org/en/regionscountries/countries/bangladesh

UNAIDS (2015) *How AIDS Changed Everything MDG 6: 15 Years, 15 Lessons of Hope from the AIDS Response*. Retrieved from http://www.unaids.org/sites/default/files/media_asset/MDG6Report_en.pdf

van den Berg, T., Schuring, M., Avendano, M., Mackenbacj, J. and Burdof, A. (2010) The impact of ill health on exit from paid employment in Europe among older workers. *Occupational Environment Medicine*, 67(12): 845–852.

van Raan, A. (2000) The interdisciplinary nature of science: theoretical framework and bibliometric-empirical approach. In P. Weingart and N. Stehr (eds.), *Practising Interdisciplinarity*. Toronto: University of Toronto Press, pp. 66–78.

Vermeulen, S. J., Campbell, B. M. and Ingram, J. S. (2012) Climate change and food systems. *Annual Review of Environment and Resources*, 37, 195–222.

von Bertalanffy, L. (1973) *General System Theory: Foundations, Development, Applications*. New York: Braziller.

Wallerstein, I. (1992) The West, capitalism, and the modern world-system. *Review*, 15(4): 561–619.

Warren, K. (1990) The power and promise of ecological feminism. *Environmental Ethics*, 12(2): 125–146.

Weiner, H. (1994) Ist das 'biopsychosoziale Modell' ein hilfreiches Konstrukt? *Psychotherapie Psychosomatik medizinishe Psychologie*, 44: 73–83.

Weingart, P. and Stehr, N. (eds.) (2000) *Practising Interdisciplinarity*. Toronto: University of Toronto Press.

Wellings, K., Collumbien, M., Slaymaker, E., Singh, S., Hodges, Z., Patel, D. and Bajos, N. (2006) Sexual behaviour in context: a global perspective. *Lancet*, 368(9548): 1706–1728.

Wilson, E. O. (1999) *Consilience: The Unity of Knowledge*. New York: Vintage Books/Random House.

Wittgenstein, L. (1999/1922) *Tractatus Logico-Philosophicus*. New York: Dover Publications.

World Health Organization (1986) *Ottawa Charter for Health Promotion*. First International Conference on Health Promotion. Ottawa, 21 November 1986. http://www.who.int/healthpromotion/conferences/previous/ottawa/en/

World Health Organization (2010) *Preventing Intimate Partner and Sexual Violence against Women: Taking Action and Generating Evidence*. Geneva: Department of Reproductive Health and Research, WHO. Retrieved from http://www.who.int/violence_injury_prevention/publications/violence/9789241564007_eng.pdf

World Health Organization (2013) *Traditional Medicine Strategy: 2014–2023*. Geneva: World Health Organization. Retrieved from http://apps.who.int/iris/bitstream/10665/92455/1/9789241506090_eng.pdf?ua=1

INDEX

absence: as absented/rectified 108, 111; as constraint 107; existence denied by philosophy 69; as ontological being 54; as presupposed by change/process 61–4
abstract universal 68
action (human): as an outcome of criticizing a belief 38; as based on values 19; as effective 93; as ethical 70; as healing 107–12; and interdisciplinary knowledge 97; as ontological being 5; as rational agency 107; as reproducing/transforming social structure 34; timeliness of 100, 105; as transformative praxis 55, 68, 107–12
actualism 31, 116, 151
ADHD (Attention Deficit Hyperactivity Disorder) 125–6, 151–2, 154
African Culture Theory (of HIV incidence) 137–9, 143–7
agency: of a medical practitioner; and structure 33–4, *Fig. 5.1*; as transformative praxis 68–70; of a woman with anorexia 107, 109–11
AIDS (Acquired Immune Deficiency Syndrome) 89, 92, 99
alcohol 104, 107, 141, 151
alethic truth 58–9
alienation 54, 156
alloplastic 70, 108
Alzheimer's disease 89: and the second enigma "What are its signs and symptoms?" 94

anorexia nervosa 4, 89, 97, *Table 10.2*; and the seventh enigma "How are we to alleviate and cure it?" 107–11
anthropology 5, 10, 97, 149
anti-imperialism *Chapter 13*, 156
antinomies 1, 4, 9, 19, *Part I*
anti-social personality disorder 104
applied critical realism 4, 45, 148
Archer, Margaret 34, 36, 43
atomism 1, 4, 12, 125, 127, 130, 151–2, 156
autoimmune condition (Derridean) 141
autoplastic 70, 108
axial rationality 154
axiological necessity 59–60
axiology of freedom (emancipatory axiology) 63–4

being 5, 54–5; as changing/processual and pre-supposing absence 61–4; as incorporating transformative praxis/human action 68–70; as meaningful 71; as prioritizing identity over difference and unity over split 72–3; as self-conscious reflexivity/agential/spiritual 70–1; as totality 65–8; as unavoidable and layered 55–60;
big bang 61
biopsychosocial approach 1, 5, 112, *Chapter 11*
BMJ (*British Medical Journal*) 100, 103
burn-out, and the second enigma "What are the signs and symptoms?" 94

CA(I)MO (model of explanation in social science) 40
cancer 116: and the second enigma "What are its signs and symptoms?" 93
capitalist economy 39
Carnivalesque Theory (of HIV incidence) 140–5, 147
categorial realism 57, 60
causal laws 29, 55, 57, 77–8
change 2, 23, 31, 37, 48, 108–9, 148; *see also* absence
cholesterol 100–3
Chomsky, Noam 38
Christian (world-view) 36, 144–7
Church, the 38–9, 42, 147
class 40, 59, 98, 109, 134
climate change 10, 17, 60, 64, 66–7, 100; and the fifth enigma "What prevents it?" 105
clinical practice 86, 113–4
clinical trials 99–100
cognitive dissonance 71
collectivism 33, 38
Collier, Andrew 49
common-sense 19
complex system 17, 114
complexity 17, 19, 49, 114, 117
concrete: detail 45, 49; object 6; phenomena 47–8, 50, 54; reality 45, 49
concrete singular 68, 95, 106, 108–10, *Fig. 10.1*, 121, 125, 145, 150
concrete universal 55, 67–8, 95, 106, 109, *Fig. 10.1*, 120–1, 125, 150
concrete universal/singular: in the ICF 120–1; and people with anorexia 108–10, *Fig. 10.1*; and people with hearing loss 120–1; and women 67–8, 145
concrete utopia 56, 69, 70, 109; as opposed to illusory utopia 56
conflict: between representations 133–5; professional 19
conjunctive multiplicity 5, 45, 51, 53, 97, 109, 138
constellation of reasons 69
consumerism 56
contradiction 2, 19, 55, 57–8, 64; in our current levels of fossil fuel use 64; in dialectic 64; as exploited by climate change deniers 66; as motivating agents 64; as not implied by advocating both epistemological relativism and ontological realism 28; not only logical 64; role in reflexive practices 71, 146; *see also* immanent critique, antinomies, TINA compromise formations, supplementarity, cognitive dissonance and theory–practice inconsistencies
correlation/causation 40, 76, 78–9, 96–7; and climate change 105; and heart disease 100–5; and HIV infection 142–3
corrigible conception 37, 80, 106
cosmic envelope 72
cosmos 69, 98
crack-user culture 142
creativity 46, 48, 49, 53, 59, 99, 124–6, 139, 151–2, 154, 155
critical realist embrace 5, 81–2
critique: of actualism 31; of conceptions held by agents 37, 80, 106; of epistemic fallacy 28, 31; as necessary for scientific work 28
crossdisciplinary understanding 2, 49, 124–5 *Fig. 12.1*, 154–5

Darwin, Charles 5, 144
de Beauvoir, Simone 144
DEA (practical problem resolution) 111–2
Derrida, Jacques 55, 71, 73n1, 81, 92, 141
diabetes 89: alleviating diabetes as retrodictive back-casting 99; diabetes as an example of the concrete universal/concrete singular 125; diabetes as a possible side-effect of statins 102; and the first enigma of healing "What is it?" 91, 93; and the third enigma "What causes it?" 96–8, *Table 10.1*
dialectic: as axiology of freedom 63–4; and contradiction 64; of science 29–30, 62–3; in society 63; as process 64; *see also* MELD, DREI(C), RRREI(C), and DEA
dialectics of Hegel, Kuhn and Bhaskar (critical realism compared) 61–2
dignity 141
disability: different explanations for 50; and mediations affecting classification 121; and participation in social life 91
disciplines: and crossdisciplinary understanding 154; education in more than one discipline 52; interdisciplinarity can lead to new disciplines 5, 153; need to complement single discipline with others 5, 10, 47–8; and process of achieving interdisciplinarity *Fig. 12.1*; tolerance of others' disciplines 50; and triple ambiguity of 11; and using different vocabulary, concepts, models 135
disjunctive plurality 5, 45, 51, 97, 109
dispositional realism 56–7, 60
drapetomania 92, 141

Index

DREI(C) (pure science of discovery) 6, 30, 45–6, 97, 102, 111–2, 132, 138–9
drinking and driving 38
dualisms 33–4: macro-dualisms 38; micro-dualisms 38–9
Durkheim, Emile 33, 35, 41

ecological constraints 66
ecological theories/claims 66–7
economics (mainstream, neoclassical) 26, 63, 154
education: for interdisciplinary practitioners *Table 2.1*, 52, 155; as neocolonialism 145; to reduce HIV infections 4, 137
educational system: French 35, 42; Norwegian 42–3
emancipation 111, 141; in critical realism 25; as dialectic 107; emancipatory discourse 59–60; emancipatory politics 110, *Fig. 10.1*; as a process of shedding 59–60; in social science 39; *see also* TTTTTT
emergence 47–9, *Table 6.1*, 53, 60, 97, 124, 149; as sometimes involving superimposition 60
emergent powers of the mind (causally efficacious reasons) 69
emotivist moral ideologies 69
empathy 88
empirical evidence 94, 103, 119, 139–40, 143–4, 147
EMR (electromagnetic sensitivity) 152; and the first enigma "What is it?" 89–91
entropy 63
environment 10, 31, 63, 70, 86, 92, 108, 116–7, 119, 141, 151
environmental science 52
epistemic fallacy 28, 31,93–4, 152
epistemological relativism 28–9, 92, 135; *see also* transitive dimension
epistemology 31, 52–8, 75–6, 80, 118, 122, *Table 12.1*, 126–7, 130, 135, 144, 150–2
ethics: ethical level of reality 50; ethical interdisciplinary behaviour 134; ethical naturalism 69; ethical thinking as concrete utopianism 56; lack of seriousness in ethical affairs 24, 69
eudaimonia 111
EURAB (European Union Research Advisory Board) 12–13, 128, *Table 12.1*
Everett, Hugh 72
evolution 5, 144; and ADHD 152
explanatory critique 70, 109
expressive-referential truth 58
extra-discursive reality 81

fact/value dichotomy (Hume's Law) 19, 38, 69; as an example of a micro-dualism in social science 33
fallibilism (knowledge is fallible) 28
feminism: and anorexia 108, 110; and HIV infection 144–7
fiduciary truth 58
Foucault, Michel 50, 81
four-planar social being 3, 34–5, *Fig. 5.1*, 125, 135
freedom 59, 63–4, 92–3, 128, 141–2
freedom from/to 107
Freud, Sigmund 71, 80, 106–7, 144
Friedman, Milton 26

Galileo, Galilei 57, 75
gay (lifestyle) 109, 144: gay culture 140, 144; gay pride 142
gender 68, 136, 139, 142–5, 152
gender-based violence: and the fifth enigma "What prevents it?" 103–5
Giddens, Anthony 34
God 71, 103, 144
green revolution 9

Hanson, Norwood 77
Harré, Rom 77
healing as praxis 107–11
heart disease (coronary) 4, 89; and the fifth enigma "what prevents it?" 100–3
hermeneutics 26, 33, 36–8, 42, 74–5, 80–1: hermeneutic moment 41; hermeneuticists were partly right 80.
Hesse, Mary 77
hidden (holistic) healing ensemble 5, 8, 87–8
HIV (Human Immunodeficiency Syndrome): epidemiology *Chapter 14*; and changing concrete universals 106; and the fourth enigma "What cures and alleviates it?" 99; and the politics of labelling people 91–2
holistic causality 2, 50, 55, 65–6, 70
Hume, David 81–2, 101, 103, 115, 122, 150
Hume's law 38
Humean: causal law 75; and empiricist scientific methodology 101, 103; Humean ontology as straight-jacket 82; ontology 27, 150; version of objectivity 122

ICF (International Classification of Functioning, Disability and Health) 6, 112–3, 116–21, *Figs 11.1* and *11.2*
ideal world of Platonic forms 25
identity 55, 62, 65, 72

ideological complex 140
ideology 76
immanent critique 24–5, 31, 75, 154; of Humean ontology/empiricist scientific method 27; as necessary for crossdisciplinary understanding 154–5
individual and collective 34–6
individualism 33, 38
induction 150; problem of, 78–9, 120; *see also* transdictive complex
instrumental approaches to prevention 100; and gender-based violence 103–5
integrative pluralism 3, 5
intentionality 70
interconnectedness of all being 70
interdisciplinarity: conditions for 51–3; definition of 10–1; antinomies of *Part I*; barriers to 14, *Table 2.1*; example of *Chapter 14*; needs disciplinarity 149; ontological case for *Chapter 6*; pessimistic, optimistic, and pragmatic approaches in mainstream literature 15–18; phases of 124, *Fig. 12.1*; practical organisation of *Chapter 12*
intradisciplinary activity 48
intransitive dimension 12, 28, 31, 42, 54, 69, 80, 90, 123–5, *Fig. 12.1*, 135
irrealist philosophy/science 18, 68–9, 82, 100

Jacob Zuma 140, 142
judgemental rationality 28–9, 42, 77, 93–4, 105, 122, 133, 143–4
Jung, Carl 35

Kant, Immanuel 26, 57, 77; as master of suspicion 80
Kantianism 19, 24, 79, 80
Kuhn, Thomas 16, 62, 87

Lancet, The 103
learning 23, 37, 87, 107, *Table 10.2*, 125, 128, *Table 12.1,* 135, 153–5
Locke, John 24

Marx, Karl 3, 41, 62, 73, 80, 110, 144
Marxism 59
masters of (the hermeneutics of) suspicion 80
master–slave 69–70, 73, 132
meaning and law 36–9
meaningfulness (of being) 5, 55, 71–2, 80
mechanisms 27–31, 47–53, *Table 6.1*, 97–8, 151–4
MELD (1M, 2E, 3D, 4L) 62, 111

metatheoretical unity 32, 52–4, 128, 148–9, 154–6
metatheory 5, 14, 18, 26, 74, 113, 117, 118, 123, 148, 149, 154; lack of 3, 11, 14
methodological individualism 153
methodological specificity *Table 2.1*, 44, 51–3
mind: dysfunctional patterns of 109; as necessary for reasoning 69, 71; of scientists 77, 79
mind–body 30–31, 33, 47
monetarism 59
monodisciplinarity 12–14, 48–9, 51, 53, 96, 110, 113, 116, 118, 124, 127, 132, 151
moral imagination 111
morphogenesis 43
multidisciplinarity 2, 4, 6, 13, 17, 47–9, 123–5, 127, 130, 144, 151, 152; and the International Classification of Functioning (ICF) 117–9
multidisciplinary-minded individuals 124
multiple-world argument 72
Mutually Agreed Tailoring: and the sixth enigma "How is it experienced?" 106

National Academy of Science (NAS) 9–12, 128, *Table 12.1*, 132
natural and social sciences compared 37, 39–41
negation 54
negative (being) 61, 63; specifically, negative values 72
negativity (2E) 54, 62, 108
Nelson Mandela 140, 142
neo-colonialism 140, 142, 145
neo-Kantians 10, 26–8, 75, 77–82
neuroscience 10
Newton, Isaac 23, 29, 58, 63, 75, 143
Nietzsche, Friedrich 71, 71, 80
Nocebo effect 85, 91
non-identity (1M) 62,72, 106
normic interactions 65
normic statements 66

ontological monovalence 61
ontological realism 28–9, 77, 92, 135
ontology 25–8, 54–73, 77, 82, 95, 97, 118, *Fig. 12.1,* 151–3, 156; in ecology 65; flat/empiricist version of 18, 27, 55, 59, 115, 122, 126–7; of general systems theory 114; ignorance about 131; of International Classification of Functioning 119; as maximally inclusive 106; in the notion of a discipline 11; as taboo 25, 82; *see also* being
oppression 70, 92, 105 140, 142–5; as power$_2$ 132

Parmenides of Elea 61
person with hearing loss (PHL) 120–1
personalism 4, 10–1; *see also* personalist moral ideology for slaves
personalist moral ideology for slaves 69
placebo effect 5, 85–7, 91, 114
Plato 25, 61
policy (social) 19, 32, 40, 67, 87, 102; and correlations 76–7, 100
polymorphous presence 2
Popper, Karl 34, 57, 66, 78, 149
positivism 33, 36, 135
postmodernism 10, 15–9, 55–7, 66, 71, 81, 92, 95, 143, 151
poverty 37, 104, *Fig. 14.1*
power: behind representation 135–6; in disciplinary hierarchies Chapter 13; as domination 132; explanatory 94; of illusions to affect us 56; of labels 92; need to use responsibly 92; in representation 133–4; as transformative capacity 132; unequal 122, 147
power$_1$ and power$_2$ 132, 134
powers: as emergent 69; as enduring 101
praxis 35, *Fig. 5.1,* 55, 62, 68, 70–1, 96, 107–11
primacy of identity (unity) over difference (split) 55, 72–4
privatisation 122
professionals 3, 6, 88, 90, 133, 136, 150, 155
psychoanalysis 144
psychology 10, 47, 52, 115, 132

Quality and Outcomes Framework (QOF) 93
quantum field 29

racism 39, 51, 72, 98, *Table 10.1*, 105, 142, 147, *Fig. 14.1*, 151, 156
reductionism 1–4, *Fig. 2.1*, 50–1, 114, 116–8, 125–7, 130, 151–3, 156
reflexivity: as auto-reflexive 70–1, 108; definition of 70; as enhanced; as the inwardized form of totality 70; in the narrative of an anorexic's life 109; as ontological 70; as a requirement of professional practice 107; in a research project 146; as spiritual 71
religious fundamentalism 70, 108
retrodiction 45–6, 51, 93, 99, 111, 127, 138; *see also* RRREI(C) and transdictive complex
retrodictive back-casting 99
retroduction 6, 29, 30, 42, 45–6, 96, 101, 105; as mode of thinking 41; as stage of research *Fig. 12.1*, 144; *see also* DREI(C) and transductive complex
retroductive: moment 82; question 41; theories 46, 103, 118, 127
revolutionary science 62, 139
Rorty, Richard 55–6
RRREI(C) (applied science) 45–6, 51, 100, 111–12, 127, 138
RRRIREI(C) (simultaneous scientific discovery and application) 46

Sartre, Jean-Paul 35
scientism 152
self-determination 107
self-realisation (dialectic of) 71; *see also* reflexivity and spirituality
seriousness 23–5, 31; and categorial realism 57; and DSM's fictive placeholders 95; and generative mechanisms and structures 66–7; and the ICF 150; and postmodernism 56; and praxis 68–9
seven enigmas of healing 3,5, 88, Chapter 10; first enigma 90–3; second enigma 93–5; third enigma 95–8; fourth enigma 98–100; fifth enigma 100–5; sixth enigma 105–7; seventh enigma 107–12
seven laminations of scale 97; as applied to diabetes *Table 10.1*
sexism 109, *Fig. 14.1*, 142, 144
slaves 69–70, 73, 92, 141
social constructionism 26, 75, 80–1, 125–6, 135, 152
social science 4, 11, 30–1, Chapter 5, *Table 12.1*
social structure 3, 33–4, 39, 41, 43, 66, 70, 108, 133, 138
speech action 31, 37, 55, 58
spiritual turn 71
spirituality 71
statins 100–3
Statistical Manual of Mental Disorders (DSM) 89; and fictive placeholders 95, 150
stratification 2–3, 29–31, 34, 58
stress (effect on humans) 86–7, 90, 94, 104, 136
structure and agency 33–4, 38
supplementarity 71

tacit knowledge/skills 38, 107
tacit ontology 26
tendency (as ontological entity) 38, 57
Thatcher, Margaret 59
theory-practice 14, 31,33, 71, 74

TINA compromise formations 59–60, 77, 81, 115, 120, 122, 136, 143
totality 2–3, 5, 24, 55, 62–5, 70–1, 108–9, 111, 125, 127
touch (human) 88
Toulmin, Stephen 77
transcendental agency 68
transcendental analysis 27; *see also* retroduction
transcendental identification in consciousness 72
transcendental objects 143
transdictive complex 150
transdisciplinarity/transdisciplinary moment 2, 11, 48, 53, 121, 124–7, 130, 153–4; contemporary anti-naturalist versions 17–9
transfactual 27, 42–3, 59, 75–7, 90, 93, 95–6, 101–5, 115, 119–20, 122–3, 126–7, 138, 143–5, 147, 150–1
transformational model of social activity (TMSA) 34, 43
transformative agency 68
transitive dimension 28, 31, 54, 58, 68–9, 80, 90–1, 106, 121, *Fig. 12.1*, 123–4, 135

truck drivers 141
trust 70, 76, 86, 92–3, 110–1, 118, 135
truth: anti-naturalistic/postmodern versions 15–9, 66, 79; critical realist version 57–9, 133; as inconvenient 96, 122; naturalistic/empiricist version 115
TTTTTT (transformed, transformative, trustworthy, totalizing, transformist and transitional praxis) 70, 107–11; *see also* praxis

UNAIDS (Joint United Nations Programme on HIV/AIDS) 138–9
unity-in-difference 123
universal solidarity 73, 154

war 37, 156 | Second World War 63
warrantedly assertable truth 58
Weber, Max 33, 71–2
WHO (World Health Organisation) 6, 117–8, 135
Wittgenstein, Ludwig von 28

Zika virus 149–50, 153

Taylor & Francis eBooks

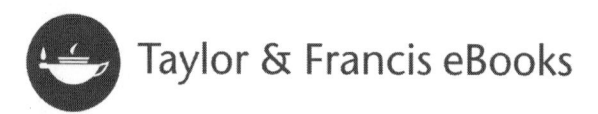

Helping you to choose the right eBooks for your Library

Add Routledge titles to your library's digital collection today. Taylor and Francis ebooks contains over 50,000 titles in the Humanities, Social Sciences, Behavioural Sciences, Built Environment and Law.

Choose from a range of subject packages or create your own!

Benefits for you
- Free MARC records
- COUNTER-compliant usage statistics
- Flexible purchase and pricing options
- All titles DRM-free.

Benefits for your user
- Off-site, anytime access via Athens or referring URL
- Print or copy pages or chapters
- Full content search
- Bookmark, highlight and annotate text
- Access to thousands of pages of quality research at the click of a button.

REQUEST YOUR FREE INSTITUTIONAL TRIAL TODAY

Free Trials Available
We offer free trials to qualifying academic, corporate and government customers.

eCollections – Choose from over 30 subject eCollections, including:

Archaeology	Language Learning
Architecture	Law
Asian Studies	Literature
Business & Management	Media & Communication
Classical Studies	Middle East Studies
Construction	Music
Creative & Media Arts	Philosophy
Criminology & Criminal Justice	Planning
Economics	Politics
Education	Psychology & Mental Health
Energy	Religion
Engineering	Security
English Language & Linguistics	Social Work
Environment & Sustainability	Sociology
Geography	Sport
Health Studies	Theatre & Performance
History	Tourism, Hospitality & Events

For more information, pricing enquiries or to order a free trial, please contact your local sales team:
www.tandfebooks.com/page/sales

Routledge — Taylor & Francis Group
The home of Routledge books

www.tandfebooks.com